Jumpstart your Metabolism

HOW TO

LOSE WEIGHT BY

CHANGING

THE WAY YOU

BREATHE

PAM GROUT

A FIRESIDE BOOK
PUBLISHED BY
SIMON & SCHUSTER

FIRESIDE
Rockefeller Center
1230 Avenue of the Americas
New York, NY 10020

Designed by Barbara M. Bachman

Manufactured in the United States of America

6 8 10 9 7

Library of Congress Cataloging-in-Publication Data

Grout, Pam.
Jumpstart your metabolism : how to lose weight by changing the way
you breathe / Pam Grout.
p.   cm.
"A Fireside book."
Includes bibliographical references and index.
1. Weight loss.   2. Respiration.   3. Energy metabolism.
I. Title.
RM222.2.G76   1998
613.7—dc21   97-36442   CIP
ISBN 0-684-84346-3

THIS BOOK IS DEDICATED TO
EVERYONE WHO REFUSED TO
GIVE UP

AND TO BOB MENDOZA,
WHO REFUSED TO GIVE UP ON ME

CONTENTS

CONTENTS

FOREWORD HO!

"OXYGEN IS THE BIG CHEESE."

SUSAN POWTER, *fitness guru*

Moses received his marching orders from a burning bush, Einstein from a star beam he imagined riding across the universe.

My marching orders were slightly less dramatic—more like a pebble that I accidentally stumbled over while going somewhere else.

The last thing I ever intended was to write a book about losing weight. Heaven knows there are enough books, enough theories, enough diets, and if you really wanted to, you could try a different one every day (probably every hour) of your life.

But then I accidentally tripped over this rather amazing discovery and suddenly had no choice. When Christopher Columbus deduced the world was round, he could have just as easily sat around in those plumed hats and tights playing tiddlywinks, but hey, he knew the earth was not flat and it was his mission to prove it.

That's sort of how I feel. I've discovered a really cheap, really convenient, and really effective way to lose weight. And it's my mission to get the word out.

It all started when somebody gave me a series of

motivational tapes by Anthony Robbins, the self-help guru whose late-night infomercials are enough to inspire a sea slug. I'd love to tell you I sat down immediately, listened to each and every tape, and suddenly became a genius, but the truth is I didn't get around to listening to most of them until a few years later.

While driving home to my mother's house for the mandatory Thanksgiving turkey, I happened to plug in a cassette in the series that talks about energy: how to get it, how to keep it. Since this was a subject I was miserably lacking in, I decided to pay attention.

At the time, I had about as much energy as a dead goldfish. I'm a single mom of a then-one-year-old. Need I say more? Between diapers, fevers, and rent payments that seemed to be due every five minutes, energy was not a word in my vocabulary. It was obviously Tony Robbins's favorite word.

Even his voice was infectious. I almost felt like stopping the car and doing a polka. He talked about energy and how the best way to get it was to breathe. Since I was presumably already breathing, I didn't think it'd be too much trouble to breathe a little more.

So I did.

Now, you've got to understand something about me. This cassette was the seventeenth in the series and so far I hadn't followed through on any of them.

But breathing was so simple, so undemanding.

Maybe I'd even follow through on his suggested twenty-one-day breathing program.

If he'd asked me to swear off chocolate or run up ten flights of stairs, now that would have been a different story. But all he wanted in return for all this boundless energy was ten deep breaths three times a day. I could fit that in between meals.

Besides, what did I have to lose? I didn't have to buy anything or go anywhere or even stick with it longer than the average lunar cycle.

Well, to make a long story short, I followed through with the breathing—all twenty-one days. And guess what?

Tony was right. I felt as if somebody finally flipped the switch. I actually had energy for the first time since my daughter, Tasman, was born. She had to be wondering what in the heck was going on. Her draggy mommy had suddenly turned into Jim Carrey. Once, I'm pretty sure I even saw her wanting to stick her finger down her throat, roll her eyes, and say, "Chill, Mom." But luckily, this was before she could speak.

The other miraculous thing that happened in those twenty-one days is I dropped ten pounds.

Like I said, losing weight was the furthest thing from my mind. Sure, I had amassed an extra ten to fifteen pounds in the process of having a baby, but after you've been in labor for seventeen hours, nothing seems too ugly or unacceptable ever again. My body seemed pretty insignificant in the whole scheme of things.

I had figured I would lose the weight later—like maybe when Tasman graduated from high school.

And then suddenly, like magic, my extra weight was gone. At first I thought I was being rewarded for finally sticking with something.

But then I remembered Louisa.

We'd met three years before at a leadership training seminar in Connecticut.

The "training" included everything from healing old parental wounds (I once had to write a joint letter to my dad, Nelson Rockefeller, and Jesus Christ) to being videotaped giving a seminar while Bob, one of the leaders, stood on his head, juggled tangerines, and did everything he could think of to distract you. But the crux of the whole program was a breathing process called rebirthing.

Without going into a lot of detail, let me just say that rebirthing is a powerful breathing exercise that you do for about an hour once a week or so. It works on a lot of stuff—mostly emotional issues that have been lodged somewhere in your body, keeping you from experiencing joy, happiness, and that movie deal with TriStar.

Louisa, who came to Connecticut from some college town in Wisconsin, was one of those people I'm sure you know. She was drop-dead gorgeous except for one small detail. Or rather large detail. She was forty pounds overweight. You know the type I'm talking about, the kind of person that everybody delights in whispering about behind her back. "Man, wouldn't she be a knockout if she'd just lose that . . . [under the breath, as if it's a dirty word] weight?"

Well, to make a long story short, in the course of the six-month training, Louisa did lose that weight. And the most remarkable thing was that she wasn't trying to lose it. She'd more or less come to terms with being what the Surgeon General calls "obese." After thirty years of being first a hefty child, then a plump teenager, and finally, an overweight adult, she had just accepted her life's fate. Oh sure, she went through a stage—if you can call twenty years a stage—where she tried all the fad diets, all the exercise gizmos, all the get-togethers of overeaters, scale watchers, etc. But by the time I met her, she had thrown her hands in the air and said, "I give up."

Then a funny thing happened. The weight that Louisa had assumed was her fate literally dropped off when she began breathing a lot.

And no, she didn't start some new exercise routine— except a few walks through the beautiful woods around Bantam Lake where she was renting a cabin. She didn't alter her eating habits. In fact, the only variable that really changed was that Louisa started breathing in more oxygen and breathing out more carbon dioxide.

At the time, everyone proclaimed it a miracle. Maybe it was the change in scenery. Maybe it was the fact she'd left her stressful job as a pharmacist. Maybe it was . . . I mean, who was going to believe that something as simple as breathing could help a person with a perpetual weight problem drop the pounds that every other scheme had failed to do.

She wasn't trying to lose weight. But it happened.

I began putting two and two together. Could it be that all the extra oxygen burns up fat?

Then I met Bobbi. I casually mentioned this crazy

theory I'd come up with about breathing and losing weight. She stared at me for a couple seconds and said, "So *that's* what happened!"

About twenty years ago, Bobbi had run across a self-help book that promised a better life in ninety days. It included a lot of exercises involving goal setting, affirmation writing, and visualizations. But it also included what Bobbi described as "this very relaxing breathing exercise," which she faithfully did every night.

In ninety days, Bobbi had met all of her goals. But something else interesting happened, as well. Bobbi inadvertently dropped twenty pounds.

"To this day, I always wondered what had happened with my weight," she said.

The mysterious cure.

People losing weight without knowing why.

Then I interviewed Gay Hendricks, a renowned therapist who has been using breathing as a transformational tool for more than twenty years.

We were talking about the physical benefits of breathing and I asked him, "Have you ever known anyone to lose weight—you know, kind of on the side?"

"Hundreds and hundreds of people," he said nonchalantly.

That did it.

I decided to launch a serious investigation. This book is what I found out.

PART ONE

THE PROMISE

"THE THING WE KNOW BEST IS
THAT OF WHICH WE ARE
THE LEAST CONSCIOUS."

SAMUEL BUTLER

1

YOU DON'T HAVE A WEIGHT PROBLEM, YOU HAVE A BREATHING PROBLEM

"IF I SHOULD HAPPEN TO FORGET, PLEASE REMIND ME TO BREATHE."

JUDY GARLAND, *to her friends, in the last days*

Grapefruit, chromium, algae. You've tried them all. You've read every diet book that's ever been written. You've aerobicized to every workout video that's ever been made. You've sent in your check, cash, or money order for every piece of exercise equipment that's ever been advertised on late-night TV.

But you're still fat.

In fact, you probably weigh more today than you did when you first noticed (how many months or years ago has it been?) that it might just be in your best interest to drop a pound or two.

Has it ever occurred to you that something is missing, that some piece of the equation has been misplaced or forgotten or maybe even purposely hidden?

It's not as if you haven't tried.

And tried some more.

Could it be that all the trying is only getting in the way?

It's ironic really. We pay Gestapo-like attention to the food we eat. We count fat grams with religious fervor. We tally calories with frenetic abandon. And yet we totally overlook the critical element that fuels our cells. We ignore the one ingredient that provides our body's energy.

It never even occurs to us to think about the amount of oxygen we consume. Yet 70 percent of the body's wastes are processed through breathing. Dr. Lawrence Lamb, a former medical consultant to the President's Council on Physical Fitness, says it's odd that we spend all this time monitoring what we take into our bodies and then completely ignore what or how it comes out. We don't even consider that the problem may be how the body is actually working.

Look at it like this: If your car's not running right, you don't keep trying different types of gasoline, different brands of motor oil. You take it to a mechanic and tune it up. You work on the heart of the problem: the system that runs the gasoline and the oil.

Good Breathing Is the Key to Weight Loss

Our bodies process three things: food, liquid, and oxygen. And while we might enjoy the food and the liquid more, it's the oxygen that actually provides the fuel that runs our body. Oxygen, through a process called oxidation, chemically changes food and liquid into energy. It's this "oxygen fire" that contracts our muscles, repairs our cells, feeds our brains, and even calms our nerves.

Not only that, but breathing is our body's chief cleansing tool. Every day, our body burns off some seven hundred billion old cells. These old cells are toxic and must be removed from our system. This is a normal, natural process of the body and nothing to worry about unless for some reason this toxic waste material is not eliminated at the same rate it's being produced. As long as we're breathing properly and getting plenty of oxygen, there is sufficient energy and the waste is easily eliminated. The problem comes when we don't take in enough oxygen.

You see, the body can store up food and liquid, but it can't store oxygen. Every minute that we are alive, we must continually provide our cells with a stream of fresh oxygen.

In fact, one of the main reasons exercise burns fat is because it increases the rate of oxygen that's delivered to your cells. When you run, for example, you increase your oxygen intake from seven or eight liters per minute to thirty-four or more liters per minute. Consequently, your body has oxygen to attend to all its energy needs.

If your body has accumulated excess fat, that means your body doesn't have the oxygen or the energy it needs to process the food you're taking in.

Take a roomful of people (any room, any people) and line them up by how much weight they could stand to lose. Creeps that are thin and lithe and obviously in shape go on one end. Those who need a personal consultation with Jenny Craig herself go on the other.

Okay, now take that same group and line them up by how much oxygen they consume. With the exception of one or two, your lineup is going to look exactly the same.

My point? People who need to lose weight don't take in their full capacity of oxygen. And while you might argue that it's the extra weight that causes them to breathe less fully than their skinny counterparts, the truth is the skimpy breathing is the catalyst for the weight problem. Not to mention, many other problems that you'll learn about in this book.

TAKE A BREATHER

....

A QUICK EXPERIMENT

S I T up straight and rest your palm on your lower belly. Okay, now take a breath. Which way did your belly move?

If your belly sucks in and flattens on the "in breath," you're breathing backward. If your belly relaxes and even expands, you are way ahead of the game. The exercises in this book will come quite easily for you.

If you look in the dictionary, the definition of food is anything your body takes in to maintain life and growth. So strictly speaking, oxygen *is* food. It's the fuel that burns the fat, the source of all energy, the ignition key that makes sure everything that bodies do gets done.

And yet we take our breathing for granted.

We certainly don't relate it to our weight problem.

Why should we? Everybody breathes. Everybody takes in oxygen.

But not everybody takes in the same amount of oxygen.

Most of us, in fact, suffer from what doctors call "futile breathing," meaning we get a quarter to a fifth of the oxygen our lungs were designed to hold. That's a major deficit. A major problem for your cells, which are trying desperately to process food, provide energy, and be the all-knowing dynamos they were meant to be.

When you don't get enough oxygen, you literally strangle your cells. It's like putting a noose around their necks, making it very difficult for them to do their job. As hard as they might try, they can't process food properly. They get bogged down, filled with sludge, and you, consequently, run out of energy.

You literally work at one fifth of your potential when you don't get enough oxygen. Your body slows down, gains weight, and becomes even more stubborn about changing.

The other startling fact is that 90 percent of us practice futile breathing in one form or another. That means nine out of ten of us aren't getting enough oxygen.

An average pair of lungs can hold almost two gallons of air. Most people settle for a measly two or three pints. It's no wonder we're getting fatter by the day.

If you're like most people, you're probably scoffing. Or

at least scratching your head. You're thinking something to the effect of, "You mean to tell me that all I have to do to lose weight is to change my breathing? That something this simple is actually going to work when every other gizmo, gadget, and pill didn't?"

The answer, quite simply, is yes. The most profound truths are often the simplest.

Let me just say right now that if you want to lose weight, you can do it by pumping up your breathing. It's not hard. It's not demanding. And you don't even have to touch your toes. In fact, you are going to feel so much better after you start breathing properly that you won't even be tempted to return to old patterns of futile breathing.

Unlike diets that require self-sacrifice, mental angst, and calculators to tally calories and fat grams, this plan is something you'll actually look forward to doing. In fact, I guarantee you'll never breathe the same again.

Another guarantee I can make is that if you bothered to pick up this book (meaning you probably have a vested interest in dropping a pound or two), you aren't breathing the way you should. If you were, you'd be too busy winning Nobel Peace Prizes or plotting your next expedition down the Amazon or at least dreaming up some new fun menu for tonight's dinner.

If you correct futile breathing patterns, you will lose weight. It doesn't matter if you are ten pounds overweight or a hundred pounds overweight. I can't guarantee that you will eventually look like Cindy Crawford, but I can guarantee that if you pump up your breathing, your health will improve and that physique that you're constantly carping about will shape up. If you practice the breathing exercises in this book, your body will automatically kick into a higher metabolism, your energy level will explode, and you can kiss your weight problem good-bye.

Congratulations! You just bought a book that will change your life forever.

TAKE A BREATHER

....

DEEP BELLY BREATHING

T H E R E are thousands of ways to breathe. But the two major categories that most of us fall into are either chest breathing or abdominal breathing. Chest breathing is inefficient and requires more breaths per minute than abdominal breathing. It also forces your heart to work harder, your blood pressure to rise, and your nervous system to pretty much stay on "red alert." So before we go any further, let's get the hang of deep belly breathing. This is the wall on which everything in this book will hang.

I like to start by lying down, relaxing.

Place a book on your stomach, right below the bottom of your rib cage. Take a deep, slow inhale through your nose, letting your belly expand like a balloon. Make sure the book is rising with each inhalation.

Now, let your abdomen fall as you exhale slowly through your nose. Press the air out, bringing that book back down.

Ahh! Now don't you feel better?

If you habitually breathe from your chest, breathing from your belly may feel uncomfortable at first. You might even feel you're reeling out of control. Trust that you're in no danger and the feeling will soon pass.

It's like learning to brush your teeth with your left hand when you've been brushing them with your right all these years. It just takes a while to get the hang of it.

Feel free to practice this breath every chance you get. You don't have to lie down. You can do it while driving to the grocery store. Just focus on breathing deeply and rhythmically into your belly, which should expand every time you inhale. Try to exhale a little longer than you inhale. This helps your body cleanse out toxins.

Eventually, deep belly breathing will become second nature and every breath you take will be fuller. Every breath will automatically deliver a fresh supply of oxygen to your once-starving cells. They're going to feel so good that they'll probably throw a party.

As often as possible, just focus on how you're breathing. Inhale into your belly. At first, it might seem like nothing much is happening, but eventually you'll really notice your belly filling up, your rib cage expanding. You'll become aware of how you breathe and how it affects every aspect of your life. Don't let this breath's simplicity fool you.

2

THE WHOLE BREATH AND NOTHING BUT THE BREATH

"HE LIVES MOST LIFE WHO BREATHES MOST AIR."

ELIZABETH BARRETT BROWNING

I don't blame you for being mad. I can't fault you for stomping your feet, pounding your chest, and screaming, "Why didn't somebody tell me this before?"

In our culture, we've become so focused on our minds that we've practically forgotten about our bodies. We're so busy paying attention to our brains that it never occurs to us to listen to what our bodies are telling us. About the only body sensations we even notice are when our backs ache or our heads pound. We certainly don't pay attention to our breathing.

Yet, breathing is the single most important thing we ever do. It's the first thing we do and the last. Go without it for three minutes and you're dead.

Breathing, quite frankly, is the most underrated activity on the planet.

Historically, this was not always the case. For many

years, the pnuema (breathing) theory dominated the healing arts. The ancient Greeks recognized the power of the breath. It's a central tenet of most Eastern religions. Know the breath, they believe, and know God. Early Hebrews used the word "breath" in context with soul. And the Bible says God created Adam by breathing life into his nostrils.

The Germans have schools devoted to breathing techniques and even here in the United States, there's a New York hospital with a twenty-four-hour hotline that dispenses tips for better breathing.

And, of course, if you've ever been involved in singing, acting, or sports, you've probably been coached on breathing.

That's what this book is all about. First, you'll learn the importance and power of the breath. Then you'll learn how to pay attention to your own breathing and, finally, how to improve it.

TAKE A BREATHER

....

NOSE VS. MOUTH?

PROBABLY the number-one question I get asked is "Should you breathe through your nose or through your mouth?" And the answer is "It depends." Some breathing techniques work best through the nose, others through the mouth. But in general, for everyday breathing, it's far better to breathe through your nose. Not only does the nose warm and moisturize the air coming in, but it directs and pulls more oxygen into the lower lobes of the lungs where there's greater potential for oxygen exchange.

There's also evidence that breathing through the nose can prevent infections and colds because the mucous membranes filter out impurities and regulate temperature and humidity.

Think of me as your own personal breathing coach. After I witnessed the power of better breathing in my own life and started talking to doctors and biochemists who verified that I wasn't crazy for believing oxygen was a miracle drug, I committed my life to spreading the gospel of the breath. Since that time, I have coached hundreds of people from Massachusetts to California.

Breathing is really pretty easy. And think of the benefits:

- *It's free.* There's nothing to buy ever again.

- *It's convenient.* You don't have to go to a gym to practice it or wear any particular clothing or, for that matter, even devote any special time to it. You can practice better breathing while driving, watching TV, or even while out on a date.

- *It's always available.* It's not as if we're about to run out of air or like some of these weird diet chemicals that you have to order secretly from some medicine man in New Mexico. Not to mention that with oxygen you don't need to go out and buy a bigger medicine cabinet.

Breathing Holds All the Answers

And that's not the best part. Learning better breathing will help with all your weight issues. As you undoubtedly know, not everybody gains weight for the same reason. Some of us have slow metabolisms; others are binge eaters. Some of us gain weight because we've developed lousy eating habits that we can't seem to shake. But the great news about learning to breathe better is it provides a way out of these common weight traps. Let's take a look at some of them and examine their relationship to breathing.

SLOW METABOLISM. Breathing changes your body physiologically. It literally transforms your body's cells from being fat storers to fat burners.

Your cells always have two choices—they either release energy or they form fat. By forming fat, a cell can process food with less oxygen. You see, it's oxygen that provides the fuel to produce the energy. Unfortunately, if you're not breathing properly, you're not delivering enough oxygen to your cells and they're forced (practically at gunpoint) to use the "low oxygen" or fat-storing processing route. That's why overweight people often feel tired. Their cells aren't releasing enough energy. It's also why football players wear those funny-looking "breath strips," specially designed to keep the nasal passages open and the oxygen flowing. They need all the energy they can get.

A study at the Lindner Clinic, a famous weight-loss facility, shows that 73 percent of all people who need to lose weight have faulty metabolisms. Why? Quite simply, they don't get enough oxygen. How could you possibly burn fat and other nutrients if you don't have enough fuel?

As you learn to breathe properly, you begin to deliver the oxygen your cells need to process food. You stimulate the enzymes that burn fat, which naturally increases your metabolic rate.

Breathing changes your body's chemistry, so once you lose weight, you can eat normally and never gain weight again.

PUTTING ON POUNDS FOR PROTECTION. Many of us gain weight to "protect" ourselves from some emotional trauma, something that might have happened back in second grade. When you breathe (particularly the connected breathing described in Part Two), you're better able to get in touch with those emotional blocks and release them.

Debbie, a client of mine, was at least sixty pounds overweight when she first started paying attention to her breathing. At thirty-one, her premarriage body was nothing but a vague memory. Every now and then, she'd get out the pictures from high school. Tish and Cindy, her best friends, didn't look that different now. She, on the other hand, was hardly recognizable.

Was that really her in the skimpy shorts and halter top?

Although she professed a desire to lose weight and bought nearly every diet book that came along, her body did little but add pounds. Which, of course, discouraged her and caused her to eat even more.

Her husband, an abusive alcoholic, constantly threatened to divorce her. He called her a fat cow and claimed she was the ugliest woman he'd ever seen. Inside, she hated him. She plotted intricate schemes to leave him, but, alas, like the diets, they were all to no avail. After all, she had the kids to think about.

When she started her breathing program and began to lose weight, an interesting thing happened. She came to realize that her weight was protection—first from her leering, abusive father and now from her husband.

Because of these long-submerged, painful feelings, Debbie's breathing program included a special, therapeutic breath called rebirthing, which I mentioned earlier. It's a type of breath that connects the inhale with the exhale (usually you pause between the two) and it can bring up a lot of old feelings. The good news is that if you keep breathing when those feelings come up, you can work through them and your breathing will return to full capacity.

Little by little, as Debbie let go of her old feelings, her breathing came back to work at full potential. It took a while, but Debbie, without any major reduction in calories, dropped all sixty pounds. She got a job and mustered the strength to leave her husband. Within a year of her divorce, she called Tish and Cindy.

"We need another group picture. Bring your halter tops."

Debbie's situation was dire, but it's clear from her story and from many others that harbored ill-will blocks the free flow of energy in your body, which, needless to say, has a giant impact on your weight. Even Nicole Kidman wouldn't look good if she were always pissed at hubby Tom Cruise. Nothing will help you drop pounds faster than letting go of unresolved emotions that are lodged in your body.

BINGE EATING AND OTHER ADDICTIONS. Binge eating has been my own personal cross. It is nothing for me to sit down and consume an entire box of Russell Stovers. My latest binges involve those cute little graham crackers shaped like teddy bears. I buy them with every good intention of giving them to my daughter for dessert—they're just her size and they're not as sugary as glazed doughnuts. But then at night when she's in bed and I'm feeling antsy, I open the box just to sample a couple—you know, just five or six. And then . . . just a couple more. And before I know it, the empty box is in the trash can and I've got this adorable three-year-old looking at me with her big brown eyes wanting to know if she can have another "gwam cwacker." You'd think the guilt alone would be enough to make me stop.

But the only thing that has ever worked is breathing. Instead of going for that second or third helping, I will sit down and take ten slow, deep belly breaths. And sure enough, the urge dissipates.

When I'm binge eating like that, I completely forget who I am, what I really want. It's almost as if I'm in a trance and don't wake up until whatever I'm eating is gone. My own personal Mr. Hyde takes over and the real me, the me who wants to be healthy and thin, disappears.

By breathing deeply, I bring my attention back to the center, back to what my real goals are. The mindless administration of food gives way to reality.

Others have given up smoking, alcohol, and many other addictions by using deep breathing.

POOR DIGESTION. A good digestive tract, as any gastroenterologist will tell you, is the cornerstone to good health. When your GI tract is working right, you digest food efficiently and distribute all the necessary nutrients to every cell.

When you don't get enough oxygen, your digestion become irregular and your body doesn't get the vitamins, minerals, amino acids, and other nutrients it needs. This is why some of us always feel hungry. Our inefficient cells are constantly starved.

Sandy, a stenographer from Reno, Nevada, called me with this very problem. Her breathing was so inefficient that, despite eating a balanced diet, she never felt satisfied. Her tissues and organs were undernourished because her digestion wasn't working the way it should. And even though she wasn't overeating, she was overweight.

I sent her some of the breathing exercises you'll find in

this book. She called a month later wanting to send me her firstborn child. To say she was overjoyed is an understatement. Not only was she enjoying her food more and actually feeling full after meals, but her extra weight had all but dropped off.

When we breathe into our chests, we release adrenaline into our systems, which slows our digestion. The energy then goes into our muscles. This is why our muscles often feel tight and we experience aches and pains. If we breathe deeply into our bellies, our autonomic nervous system goes "off alert," our muscles relax and our digestive system kicks back in. Scientists claim deep breathing increases gastrointestinal peristalsis (the involuntary muscle contractions of your intestines), blood flow, and food absorption.

A yoga teacher I know of hosts breath luncheons for her students. During the meal, they simply observe how they're breathing. You'll find that if you loosen up your abdomen and stomach while you're eating, you'll eat less, enjoy your food more, and digest your food better.

CAN'T STAND TO EXERCISE. There's a very good reason that many people would rather slit their wrists in a warm bath than exercise. Most of us take shallow breaths when we exercise, only filling the upper two lobes of our five-lobed lungs. The nerve receptors in the upper chest stimulate the body's "fight or flight" mechanism by producing a buildup of stress chemicals and fighting hormones. The body actually thinks it's in a state of emergency. In other words, exercise is not a pleasant sensation. When we breathe deeply and rhythmically into our bellies, we stimulate the nerve receptors that calm and regenerate the body. Exercise with proper breathing actually becomes fun. It becomes something we enjoy, something we'd actually choose to do.

EATING FOR COMFORT. Many of us use food the way Linus uses his blanket. Eating signals the pituitary gland to release endorphins. These natural chemicals slow and smooth out the digestive process, but they also make you feel so good that you sometimes want to eat more.

Lisa was only ten pounds overweight when I first met her. Not a bad record—especially when you figure she gained sixty pounds while pregnant with little Denny, her then-three-year-old. But, oh those ten pounds. According to Lisa, she'd tried everything—even bought a pair of those silly lose-weight-while-you-sleep pants.

But those last ten pounds refused to budge. Her main problem was that, during her first year at home with Denny, she'd fallen prey to the soap opera and bonbon syndrome. In other words, she was hopelessly addicted to sugar.

Lisa learned to fight the sugar cravings through breathing. Whenever that urge would arise (and at first it was every ten minutes), Lisa would consciously breathe deeply instead of giving in to her cravings.

Breathing, when done properly, actually signals the brain to release endorphins in your body the same way eating does. Endorphins, as you probably know, are natural drugs that make you feel good. Before she started breathing, Lisa was using the sugar to release the endorphins.

So by self-administering oxygen, she was able to "just say no" to all the sugar she'd been mainlining for three years. Quite naturally, she dropped those last ten nasty pounds. Last I saw her, she was still thin, and while she did succumb to a hot fudge sundae every now and then, she had been able to combat her overpowering sugar addiction by breathing.

"The only problem now," she told me, "is I'm addicted to oxygen. I have to do my breathing exercises or I feel like I'm dancing on one leg."

THE INVISIBLE BODY. This syndrome is the major hurdle for most people wanting to lose weight. We don't listen to our own bodies. We certainly look at them, despising the image we see in the mirror, but we don't really pay attention to what they're telling us.

This "invisible body" syndrome is our primary screwup.

In fact, the absolute greatest benefit of proper breathing is it puts you back in touch with your body. The problem with most weight-loss programs is they advocate someone *else's* remedies. Maybe your body doesn't like the exercises of the Royal Canadian Air Force.

With breathing, you learn to listen to your own inner wisdom, you find the answers that are within yourself. Your body has been trying to get through to you for a long time. It's constantly tapping at your door, clearing its throat with its polite "ahems."

Your body knows how to heal itself. It knows exactly how to lose weight. However, when you keep trying one diet after another, you give your body the message that you don't trust it.

Your body is quite miraculous. In fact, it wants to be thin even more than you do. And it knows perfectly well how to get that way, but it can't seem to get your attention long enough to fill you in. Instead, it's forced to constantly fight as you wage war again and again with another diet.

Consequently, you're totally cut off from the one ally, the only ally, that can really help.

By practicing deep, slow breathing, you will get to know your body. You'll learn to tune in to the wisdom it has to offer. This one change will revolutionize your life. Pay attention to your body, heed its plea, and let go.

Yes, the answer to whatever weight issue ails you is as simple as changing the way you breathe.

I'm not asking you to take my word for it.

All I ask is that you try it. What do you have to lose? It doesn't take long—certainly not more than fifteen minutes a day—to try the exercises. If you don't notice any positive changes in your life, you're certainly welcome to resume your old ways of breathing, to throw this book in your nearest trash can. But I'd be willing to bet dollars to sugar-free doughnuts that your life is about to take a dramatic and exciting new turn.

Breathing will set you free. Forever.

TAKE A BREATHER

....

GEOMETRIC BREATHING

W H E T H E R you visit a mainstream exercise instructor in Des Moines, Iowa, or a Pranayama guru in California, you'll probably encounter these two basic exercises, which nearly every expert swears by.

TRIANGLE BREATHING. It is the simplest breathing exercise you can do, wherever you happen to be. You don't need a leotard or a tape or a perky, bouncy fitness expert to lead you.

1. Simply inhale through the nose for a count of four.

2. Hold the air in your lungs for a count of four.

3. Exhale through the nose for a count of four.

Not only does this assure you of a complete and rounded breath, but it forces you to focus purely on the act of breathing—invaluable if you're trying to unclutter your mind to concentrate on a race, a business meeting, or whatever shrieking reality you find yourself in. Visualizing a triangle as you count (mentally "moving" from point to point) will also help you keep your rhythm as you relax.

If you do this for three or four minutes at a

stretch, you'll lower your stress level, both mental and physical. The old ticker will thank you for it, and the lungs will finally get a well-deserved break from the sporadic and tension-fraught air-gulping to which you've been subjecting them.

SQUARE BREATHING. Yes, you math experts out there, this is the same basic exercise as the triangle with an added hold of four counts after the exhalation, pausing before taking in your next breath. This further increases the level of oxygen in the lungs and therefore in the bloodstream.

(Incidentally, there isn't an endless array of geometrically named exercises—nothing, for example, called "rhombus breathing.")

As you begin to become conscious of how you should actually be breathing all the time, this awareness will begin to filter into your daily life. You will begin to notice when you're not breathing normally and when your breaths are coming in short gasps from the chest or when your mind is racing. You will automatically begin deep belly breathing, which will immediately relax you and calm your mind.

3

TAKE OUT YOUR PENCIL— A TEST TO SEE IF YOU HAVE A BREATHING DISORDER

"BREATHING IS UNQUESTIONABLY THE SINGLE MOST IMPORTANT THING YOU DO IN YOUR LIFE. AND BREATHING RIGHT IS THE SINGLE MOST IMPORTANT THING YOU CAN DO TO IMPROVE YOUR LIFE."

SHELDON SAUL HENDLER, M.D.,

biochemist, and author of The Oxygen Breakthrough

If you're like most people, the idea of altering your weight with your breath is intriguing. (Think of all the money you could save on diet books.)

But at the same time, you have a lot of resistance. You're not convinced that you really have a "breathing problem." Your aunt Ida is the one with the breathing problem. She's the one with the inhaler and the cloth mask.

Okay, perhaps "problem" is a bit strong. I prefer to

think of the old brain analogy. You know the one that says we humans use only 10 percent of our brain power. I know you've heard this before. The 10 percent brain power maxim is part of our planetary consciousness— like hot dogs at baseball games or grandmas going goochy-goochy over babies. I don't recall if it was Benjamin Franklin or Ralph Waldo Emerson or Mrs. Boston, my fourth-grade teacher, who passed down the old brain maxim, but I believe it also applies to our breathing. All of us greatly underutilize the possibilities.

Tom Goode, managing director of the International Breath Institute, an organization dedicated to spreading the good news about breathing, estimates that 90 percent of the American population exhibits restricted breathing patterns.

We just don't know it.

Take this short quiz to see if well . . . maybe . . . should we say . . . to see if your body is respirationally challenged?

1. *Stand up. Place your right hand on your chest and your left hand right below your belly button. Now, take a normal breath. Which hand went up higher?*

If it was your left hand, give yourself 10 points. If it was your right hand, you get 0 points, but don't panic. There are seven questions left.

2. *How would you rate your metabolism compared to most of the people you know?*

If it seems higher than the average Joe—meaning you can eat a lot more than most people can without gaining weight—give yourself a 10. If you seem about average, tally up a 5. If your metabolism is obviously lower than most of the people you know (you can't even walk by a pastry shop without gaining weight), give yourself a 0.

3. *How well can you express your feelings?*

Can you cry when you're sad? Admit anger when the dunce in the car ahead of you cuts you off on the freeway? Do you freely express your love to the people you know?

You may be wondering what this has to do with your breathing. It's a well-documented fact that when people attempt to withhold their emotions, they also hold their breath. It's the most effective way possible to keep your emotions from coming out. While this may be handy in some situations, it plays havoc on your breathing mechanism.

So if you feel you are extremely expressive with all your emotions, give yourself a 10. If you're about average, you get a 5. And for those of you who'd rather get run over by Shaquille O'Neal than to let anyone know what you're feeling, chalk up a 0.

4. *How are you at stairs?*

If you can easily walk up two flights of stairs without feeling winded, give yourself a 10. If you can easily make it up the stairs, but your breathing definitely gets a lot harder, give yourself a 5. If you feel like lying down and taking a nap every time you mount a couple of flights, mark down 0.

Don't despair if you're getting lots of 0's. Remember that just means you're a prime candidate for this book and you're about to learn some techniques for resetting your metabolism and transforming your life.

5. *Find a watch with a second hand. Count how many breaths you take per minute. This may take a few tries. For one thing, you're paying attention to something you usually ignore. It's important to relax and note the natural rhythm of your breathing.*

If it's between four and seven, give yourself a 10. If it's eight to fourteen, you get a 5. If you take more breaths than fourteen, give yourself a 0.

6. *Which of the following song lyrics best describes your life:*

a. "Sunshine, lollipops, and rainbows everywhere" **(10 points)**

b. "Ho hum, di dum dum dum" **(5 points)**

c. "Blue, blue, my world is blue" **(0 points)**

Again, you may be wondering what in Sam Hill this has to do with breathing. Scientists have discovered that people who don't get enough oxygen often fight depression. And from my experience, it's pretty difficult to stay down in the dumps once you fully oxygenate your body. Your breathing is a near-perfect representation of your willingness to dive into life.

If you only breathe about half of what's possible, you're probably settling for about half of what life has to offer. If you breathe with gusto and take in every last ounce of oxygen that's available to you, you undoubtedly approach life the same way.

One of my first breathing coaches pointed out to me that breathing has to do with trust. If you trust that people are good, that life is working on your behalf, you tend to breathe fully. On the other hand, if you're not quite sure whether or not to trust life, you probably hold your breath.

7. *How is your weight compared to say Susan Powter?*

If you strike a remarkable resemblance, you must have been coerced into reading this book, but give yourself a big 10, not to mention a pat on the back. If your weight is between five and ten pounds above where you'd like it to be, give yourself a 5. If you're more than ten pounds overweight, give yourself a 0.

8. *Which statement best describes your energy level?*

a. I have so much energy it's hard for me to sit down and even take this silly test. Okay, give yourself a 10.

b. I wish I had more energy, but I'd hardly call myself a sloth. You guessed it. 5 points.

c. My energy level reminds me of a sloth's sex life. It takes him two days to get worked up enough to even have it. Give yourself a 0.

Okay, How Did You Do?

80 POINTS. If you received a perfect 80 points, you're an Einstein of breath. You might as well chop this book up for firewood. Or better yet, write your own.

60 TO 79 POINTS. Your breathing is remarkably better than the average breather. In fact, you're already firmly aware of the power of the breath and I won't have

to do any talking to convince you to breathe even more. You're sold. Read on, O breathing warrior.

40 TO 59 POINTS. Hey, what can I say? You're halfway there. You don't need Aunt Ida's inhaler and you probably don't have to worry about keeling over at Bloomingdale's, but it certainly would behoove you to breathe a little deeper. Take ten deep breaths and meet me in Chapter 4.

39 OR LESS. You're probably hanging your head, wondering if you shouldn't just go out for a loaf of bread and never come back. Nothing could be further from the truth. In fact, you're the one who should be cheering. You've just unlocked the secret to many of your life's ailments. As you read this book and practice the breathing exercises, you are going to discover radical changes in your life. Radical *good* changes. Congratulations! You may now thumb your nose at those people in the other categories.

TAKE A BREATHER

DARTH VADER HAS THE RIGHT IDEA

IT'S common to hear the advice "take a deep breath." But how often have you been advised to take a deep exhale? On every exhale, you want to squeeze out as much air as possible. Your lungs are the body's main excretory organ. When you don't get rid of all that stale air, you leave poisons in your system that slow your body down. So from now on, the most important component of your newfound breathing practice is to get rid of all that old air that's probably been sitting at the bottom of your lungs since eighth grade. Among other things, dead air is a breeding ground for germs, not to mention that it can cause halitosis.

Remember Darth Vader in *Star Wars*? Remember how he sounded when he breathed? You want to tighten your throat on the exhale and pretend you're Darth Vader. This constriction of the throat activates your stomach muscles to tighten, which also helps push out that leftover air.

4

HOW YOUR BREATH BECAME
A NINETY-POUND
WEAKLING

"HE WHO HALF BREATHES, HALF LIVES."

ANCIENT EASTERN PROVERB

Remember when you were a kid and you were mad at your mom for not letting you bite holes in the middle of your bologna and cheese sandwich and you decided to "show her" by holding your breath?

Well, the reason she didn't exactly fall all over herself patting you on the back, abandoning the meat loaf she was mixing to desperately revive you, is because she knew that by the time the second hand went around on her watch, your reflexes would kick in and override your stubbornness.

Because while most of us can go something like two weeks without food (I couldn't, but those explorers who get lost in blizzards supposedly can) and two days without water, we can only go about three minutes without oxygen (and after about two minutes, there is usually irreparable damage to vital organs, including the brain).

Breathing is so important that it's not something we have to remember to do. If it were left up to us, some of us would forget it the way we forget to wear non-holey underwear (you know, in case of car wrecks) or misplace it along with the phone bill. Luckily, breathing isn't a task that requires us to make a conscious effort. Too risky. Instead, it's automatic.

That's the good news. The not-so-good news is that even though breathing is impossible to override, it's also very easily disturbed.

Every time you get upset, you hold your breath—not a lot, but just enough to decrease the intake of oxygen. Think about those times when you were really sad and felt like crying, but because you were in your boss's office or in the third pew of the church at your cousin's wedding, you were too embarrassed to let it all hang out. By holding your breath, you managed to hold back the tears.

Whenever you're scared, your breathing tends to speed up and become shallow.

When a person's physical or emotional state changes, breathing changes right along with it. And interestingly enough, a change in breathing patterns also affects your emotions. Try this little demonstration. Sit erect, raise your shoulders and collarbone, and lean forward. Now try to inhale. Feels a little scary, huh?

The connection between breathing and emotions is no big secret. It's been known for thousands of years and is being rediscovered every day in medical and psychology labs all over the world.

Even the tiniest mood change is reflected in your

breathing. As you probably know, there have been whole books written about body language and how you can tell what a person is feeling by the way he holds his body. Even better at reflecting telltale emotions is a person's breathing patterns. In fact, in neurolinguistic programming, psychologists advise people who want to create rapport to first copy each other's breathing patterns. So next time you're trying to woo a date or wow a boss, just pay attention to how he or she is breathing and follow it in rich detail. Each person has his or her own unique breathprint—much like a fingerprint.

Unfortunately, most of us are completely oblivious to our signature breathprint. Because breathing is something we don't have to concentrate on, it's usually placed on the priority list somewhere down with clipping our toenails. And since we don't pay attention, we don't even realize that we oftentimes "breathe backward," as the famous opera tenor Luciano Pavarotti likes to say.

Take the average person and ask him to take a deep breath. More than likely, even if he's a trained topflight athlete, he'll suck in his belly, puff out his upper chest and hunch his shoulders up to his ears like Nixon during the Watergate period. The great majority of us don't take full breaths. We settle for teensy, tiny, wimpy breaths. Which would be okay, except that by refusing full expression of our lungs, we're also saying no to full expression of our emotions, our potential, and, for that matter, our lives. Not to mention that it makes us gain weight.

Let's assume you're one of the nine out of ten who isn't

breathing fully. You're probably wondering what happened. Why me?

Before you panic and head for the nearest razor blade, rest assured that your breathing can be adjusted. It's just a matter of paying attention and making your breathing a priority. Take it off the toenail list and put it up with eating and sleeping. It's that important.

At any time, your breathing is somewhere along a continuum. At best, it's complete and full, coming into your lungs in a deep, slow, rhythmical pattern. The other end of the spectrum features rapid, shallow breathing that sounds something like a panting dog.

There are many reasons why people shut down their breathing. Your reason is as unique to you as your breathprint.

Some of the more popular reasons:

1. CULTURAL CONDITIONING. From the time we were able to wobble around on two legs, we were trained to stand with our shoulders back, our chests out. And while such military poses are terrific at impressing obnoxious drill sergeants, they do nothing to promote good breathing. Full breathers stick out their guts and go for it. Such cultural uniforms as mini-skirts, stretch pants, and other tight clothes are another deterrent to breathing with gusto.

TAKE A BREATHER

THE PROBLEM WITH "SUCKING IT IN"

YOU'RE probably not thinking about good breathing as you reach for that slinky black skirt, but clothes—and even shoes—can hinder your ability to breathe efficiently. Beware of:

- Clothes that pinch your waist or squeeze your stomach
- Clothes that are too small
- Tight belts or waistbands
- Tightly knotted scarves or neckties
- High heels, shoes that pinch
- Tight bras or underwear
- Girdles, corsets, "control top" anything

2. EMOTIONAL REPRESSION. A lot of us quit breathing fully because we didn't want to feel our feelings. We held our breath to hide from a lot of things we were taught not to do—like get angry, cry in public, or scream at our parents.

The only problem is that while holding our breath and breathing shallowly can effectively shut down our feelings, it can't get rid of them. They just get locked somewhere in the muscles of our bodies. Our guts get knotted with anxiety. What's worse, they also shut down those feelings of joy and spontaneity.

If you're not breathing properly, you probably haven't experienced anything like joy or bliss for a long time. And let me guess, you justify this emotional repression with an excuse like, "Hey, I'm an adult, I'm not supposed to feel those things."

Well, I've got news for you. If you start breathing in more oxygen, you're going to feel joy and, yes, even bliss. Shutting down your breath is shutting down your life. Take a deep breath right now! Don't you feel better!

3. TRAUMA. Whenever we experience a threat to our well-being, we immediately generate energy to meet the threat. Our hearts beat faster and we prepare to "take flight." This response was particularly useful back in the Stone Age when the Fred Flintstones of the day ran into wild, foaming boars or Dinos that hadn't been domesticated yet.

And while, yes, breathing does resume its natural state once the fear or the stress is gone, it tends to not quite go back to its optimum state—especially if you get scared or stressed a lot.

When the emotional wind gets knocked out of us, it often feels safer to shut down the gut a little bit, to breathe just a little less fully.

So unless you've had a perfect life, you probably aren't breathing fully. If you came from a totally functional family and your mom and dad and every man or woman you ever loved always loved you back and if you never were scared of heights or Son of Sam or anything like that, maybe you don't have a breathing problem. But so far, I haven't met anyone who had a perfect emotional batting average.

4. PHYSICAL PROBLEMS. Just check with your local lung specialist for the long list of illnesses that affect breathing. The few I can think of off the top of my head are asthma, pneumonia, bronchitis, laryngitis, tuberculosis, allergies, chronic sinusitis, and common colds. Seemingly unrelated diseases such as chronic fatigue, arthritis, and epilepsy are also contributors to disordered breathing. In fact, hooray for the doctors who are starting to prescribe breathing exercises to help counteract some of these "unrelated" diseases. Even things like bad posture, snoring, and slumping can affect the way you breathe.

5. BIRTH. Think about it. You're comfortably ensconced in your mother's womb. The environment is cozy—perfect temperature, plenty of food, no chance of a sunburn, the music of your mother's heartbeat a constant comfort—and then wham! One day, you're pushed violently out into a room of bright lights, loud voices, and nurses wearing weird surgical masks. And if that wasn't bad enough, that strange doctor whose only job, as you recall, was to thrust weird instruments your way reels back and swats you on the behind. It's enough to take anyone's breath away. At least it's not a very reassuring way to prompt your first breath.

There's a whole school of breathwork that focuses on nothing but overcoming the traumatic breathing patterns you picked up at birth. Dr. Frederick LeBoyer, a French obstetrician, even wrote a bestselling book called *Birth*

Without Violence that encourages mothers to bear babies in a completely different manner. Studies have shown that babies who were born the LeBoyer way have less restricted breathing patterns and consequently healthier, more vibrant lives.

6. SMOKING. Enough said.

TAKE A BREATHER

....

AN ASSIGNMENT

IN *The Breathing Book,* expert Donna Farhi writes: "Breathing affects your respiratory, cardiovascular, neurological, gastrointestinal, muscular and psychic systems and also has a general effect on your sleep, your memory, your energy level, and your concentration."

And you're still wondering if it's important to practice proper breathing?

Your assignment for the next few days is to notice other people's breathing patterns. Notice how their emotions are reflected in their breath. When people are angry, for example, notice how their breath is short and jerky. When they're scared, notice that their breath picks up speed. That's why actors trying to demonstrate certain emotions often start with how their character breathes. Just pay attention for a couple days. See what you can learn.

5

DIETS ARE RED HERRINGS

"NO FOOD OR DRUG WILL EVER DO FOR YOU WHAT A FRESH SUPPLY OF OXYGEN WILL."

TONY ROBBINS, Unlimited Power

It doesn't take a rocket scientist to figure out that diets don't work. If they did, why does every adult American weigh, on an average, eight pounds more than they did ten years ago? If diets delivered on all the promises they made, why are a third of us—not just fat—but obese?

And the even more pertinent question, as far as I'm concerned, is why do we persist in depriving and disciplining ourselves in the name of diets when they obviously suck sewer slime. Think of it like this. If you went to collect your paycheck and your boss said, "Sorry, but we've decided not to pay you this week," would you keep working at that job, week after week, hoping that someday he'll have a change of heart?

Yet, this is exactly what we do when we attempt to start yet another diet. Some of us put ourselves through this process of pain and punishment on a regular basis—every Monday or every New Year's Day or every time we see a new diet touted in the women's magazines. And while all this suffering would be worth it if we were guaranteed a body like Pamela Anderson, the grim statistic is this: 95 percent of us regain the weight we lose from dieting. Instead of Pamela Anderson, we end up with our own bodies—only fatter.

Nick Russo, a New Jersey real estate investor who had spent three decades struggling to lose 360 pounds, even went so far as to offer a $25,000 reward to anyone who spotted him going off his diet. He actually hung "wanted" posters of himself eating at his favorite restaurants. He lost 114 pounds, gained back 80, upped the ante to $100,000 and lost 40 more. But today, five years later, he's back to 310 pounds.

A friend of mine was moaning about her boyfriend's alcoholic behavior. Every time she called, she was disappointed because he'd gotten drunk and forgotten about a dinner party she'd invited him to or gotten drunk and spent the money they were going to use for Elton John tickets or gotten drunk and . . . you get the picture. I finally asked her, "Why do you persist in expecting sane behavior from an insane person? It's like going to a shoe store to buy milk. You can go back time and time again, but that shoe store is never going to sell milk." Likewise, her alcoholic boyfriend is never going to act the way she wants him to. And those diets you keep trying are never going to permanently take the weight off.

We've been brainwashed into believing that dieting keeps us slim. If we can just refrain from eating that extra piece of pie, if we can just follow the recipes in the back of this book or that book, if we can just deprive ourselves of enough calories, our weight will magically disappear and we'll all live happily ever after. Not only that, but Prince Charming will probably pull up on a white stallion and our bosses will hand us a six-figure raise.

Where did we get this erroneous notion? It's certainly not from experience. I dare you to name three people who have lost weight on a diet and not gained it back.

What's the number-one thing you think about when you start a diet? Food, particularly fattening food that you can't wait to eat again when the grueling ordeal is finally over. Even the spelling of the word should give us a clue. Who wants to do anything that has the word "die" in it? Psychologically (not to mention physiologically), diets are never going to fly. They go against human nature.

Even though we look to diets for answers, we subconsciously put up our dukes, become defiant. On the outside, we're saying, "I want to be thin. I'm going to quit eating waffles and French toast for breakfast." But that little voice inside us, that sneaky, tiptoeing subconscious, crosses its arms across its chest and says, "Like hell I will."

TAKE A BREATHER
....
SUCCESS STORY

TONY is tall, dark, and handsome, the kind of guy who could have made that Diet Coke commercial. You know, the one where all the secretaries gather at eleven-fifteen to watch the construction worker take off his shirt and guzzle the Diet Coke. But Tony wasn't happy with his weight—not so much because he didn't look good (believe me, he did), but because he felt the thirty extra pounds were sucking down his energy. As he describes it, he could barely drag himself out of bed—even after the third slam dunk of the snooze alarm.

Tony wasn't about to start haphazardly trying any old diet that came along. He'd seen enough people lose weight only to gain it back. No, Tony was a smart cookie. He decided to do some research before even attempting his weight-loss program. He went to the library. He consulted with doctors. He took nutritionists out to lunch.

And, like most of us, he came to the realization that there are more theories on weight loss than there are on child-rearing. That didn't dissuade him. He just kept looking. Only instead of so-called "experts," he went straight to the horse's mouth, straight to the people who had not only lost weight, but who had managed to keep it off as long as five years later. In other words, people who had changed their body chemistries for good.

And do you know the one element that all the successful weight-loss programs had in common?

Oxygen, pure and simple.

Tony, of course, knew a good thing when he saw

it. He proceeded to follow a deep-breathing regimen that he concocted out of all the theories put together and he dropped twenty pounds in thirty days. Ten years later, he's still a candidate for a Diet Coke commercial, still smart, and because he's still breathing and exploding with energy, he's the number-one self-help guru in America. His name is Tony Robbins and if you want to hear more about how he used the breath to lose weight and achieve great energy levels, check out his books and tapes.

As Carlos Castaneda said in *The Second Ring of Power,* "People love to be told what to do, but they love even more to fight and not do what they are told."

I know every time I made a conscious effort to lose weight through dieting, I found myself doing just the opposite. The classic story is when my old roommate, Kitty, and I decided to challenge ourselves to a competition. Whoever lost ten pounds first would buy the other a new dress. We dutifully got out the scales (what self-respecting woman doesn't own at least one set of scales?), weighed in, and wrote our respective starting weights on our calendars. It was a Monday. By the next Monday, Kitty had gained three pounds and I had gained four.

Before you get any ideas, let me come clean right here and now. I have never had much of a weight problem. I've fluctuated ten or twenty pounds, but because I'm tall, I was always able to hide the extra weight. In fact, my favorite joke about weight loss is that people have been wasting their time trying to lose weight. Instead, they should try to grow a couple of inches.

But, because I grew up in America when Twiggy and all those other toothpicks were the rage, I couldn't escape the compulsion and the desire to wage many a diet. In high school, I shunned soft drinks and chocolate (this also had something to do with Clearasil not working). In college, I took up jogging and when I was a twenty-something professional, I tried everything from Dexatrim to picturing my food with gross, slimy worms crawling out of it. This was a diet my sister read about in some teen magazine.

Which brings up another point. There are more theories on dieting than there are on the Kennedy assassination. One diet swears by loading up on protein. The next says, "Oh, horror, avoid protein at all costs. Focus instead on carbs." And still another claims, "Eat whatever you want, just make sure you wash it all down with papaya."

Wading through the mire of diet ideas is enough to drive a sane person straight to the edge.

The Skinny on Diets

Even worse than the psychological land mines that come with dieting are the physical problems. Dieting on a regular basis actually resets your body's metabolism to a lower level. One study showed that dieters, after just three days of decreasing their calorie intake, also decreased their basal metabolism (that's your metabolism when you're not doing anything) by 20 percent.

Your body, you'll hear me say over and over again, is an extremely wise and efficient machine. When it doesn't get the food it's used to, red lights go off and it thinks, "Famine ahead, better stock up." So it slows down your metabolism and starts storing fat.

So not only does dieting not work but it makes your body even more prone to fat than it was when you started the diet in the first place.

Dieters are literally draining themselves—not only physically, but mentally (self-esteem suffers every time you attempt a diet and fail), spiritually (worshiping calories and fat grams replaces love and joy), and financially.

I don't know how much you've contributed to this alarming statistic, but every year dieters in America spend $33 billion. If we devoted that same amount to the national deficit, we could probably pay it off in a couple of years. And if that doesn't get you in the gut, think of this: If you had $33 billion, you could spend a million dollars a day for eighty years and still have millions to leave to your favorite charity. In other words, that's a lot of moola.

And again, if diets worked, all that money might be worth it. But dieting does not and will not ever work.

At best, it's a temporary fix. So if you want a temporarily skinny physique, by all means, find another diet, start another regimen of deprivation and pain. But if you'd like a physique that is permanently slim and trim, you've come to the right place.

This book is not going to ask you to count any calories or tabulate any fat grams. For that matter, it's not even going to ask you to do any sit-ups—although its author would certainly applaud if you decided to do so.

Skinny People Are Different *Inside* Their Bodies

What this book does is address the issue that Dr. Lawrence Lamb, former adviser to the President's Council on Physical Fitness, brought up in 1983. "It's incredible that so much attention has been given to decreasing calories while so little has been given to influencing calories out."

In other words, it's ironic that we spend so much time thinking about dieting and so little time thinking about how to better process the food we eat. That's what this book is about. It's about changing the way you process food. It's about changing your body from the inside out.

Your body is a nonstop janitor. In its never-ending pursuit of health, it continuously cleanses itself of unnecessary wastes. The faster your body is able to eliminate dead cells, worn-out blood proteins, old tissues, and various other metabolic wastes, the healthier you are.

This job is a piece of cake when you're breathing up to par, but when you're not getting enough oxygen, your body is unable to eliminate the toxins as fast as it's supposed to. Remember 70 percent of all wastes are processed through your breathing.

And when you don't get rid of the toxins, you gradually accumulate extra waste and, hey, it has to go somewhere. Your body has little choice but to deposit those wastes in fat cells.

This wouldn't be so bad except it also ties up your energy. You need this energy.

Your body works an awful lot like a car. Your food, like gas, oil, and other fuel, is made up of hydrocarbons. Combine it with oxygen and energy is ignited. In fact, the phrase "burning off fat" is not as far-fetched as it sounds. Without oxygen, there can be no flame, no heat, no getting rid of all those darn calories.

Think of it like this. If you bought a brand-new Ferrari (I'd settle for a new Jeep Cherokee myself), you probably wouldn't buy the cheapest gasoline you could find. Instead, you'd buy the best fuel you could find. And you'd make sure you filled up the tank.

That's what the exercises in this book will do for you. They'll make sure you're getting the very best fuel at the very best price.

Dr. Jack Shields, a highly respected lymph system specialist from Santa Barbara, California, put cameras inside people's bodies to see what stimulated the removal of toxins. You guessed it? Deep diaphragmatic breathing. He found that deep belly breathing can multiply the pace at which your body eliminates toxins by as much as fifteen times.

Kind of enough to make you want to take a deep breath.

TAKE A BREATHER

SPINE LIMBERER

ONE of the main reasons good breathers look younger than panters is because their spines are limber. Your rib cage, which houses your lungs, is attached to your spine, so every time you inflate your lungs fully you give your spine a much-needed workout. And any doctor can tell you that a limber spine is the key to longevity and good health. Here's a good exercise to try.

1. Lie on your back.

2. Start by exhaling through your nose.

3. As you exhale, stretch your spine, tipping your tailbone in the air. The tipping of the tailbone will also flatten your stomach, which squeezes out stale air.

4. When you've squeezed out as much air as you can, relax and let the inhale come naturally. At first, it will feel as if you're not getting air in. But trust me—the vaccum effect from the strenuous exhale will draw plenty of air in.

5. Repeat the series twelve times.

6

WHY BREATHING WILL BLOW YOU AWAY

When I first discovered that you could lose weight by breathing more, questions began whirling through my mind like the Tasmanian Devil.

How could something so simple be so effective? How could something so effective be overlooked? Surely, in a century of weight-loss obsession, somebody somewhere would have made the connection before. I mean, if people can come up with sexy pineapple diets (eat one twice a week, say the Danish authors, and not only will you lose weight but your sexual stamina will explode) and wine diets (the idea, I suppose, is that if you imbibe enough dry wine with your meal, you'll pass out before you can get to the rich, fattening stuff), surely someone would have figured out that you can drop pounds by pumping your body with oxygen.

Well, I soon learned that someone did—namely the

founders of aerobic exercise. Aerobics, if you remember, is a term that means "exercise with air." Although we've been "exercising with air" ever since the first caveman lustily chased his bride-to-be through the canyon, the term wasn't actually coined until the mid-sixties, when Dr. Kenneth Cooper discovered that oxygen is the key to making our bodies work better.

The other major branch of exercise is anaerobic exercise, which is exercise that doesn't require oxygen—or at least not more than you'd use sitting on a couch reading *The Bridges of Madison County*. Weight lifters, bodybuilders, and other studly, muscle-bound types focus on anaerobic exercise, which, as you can tell from looking at pictures of Arnold Schwarzenegger, doesn't exactly inspire frail, thin physiques.

Aerobic exercise, which includes such activities as jogging, dancing, and running up and down the stairs trying to find your car keys, does. People discovered if they would bounce, jump, twist, and run until they were panting like a lapdog they could lose weight. But what they failed to realize was that it was the extra oxygen that really did the work. Sure, the extra muscles helped. Lean muscle burns through fat a whole lot faster than flab. But the bottom line to their success was they transformed their bodies from being fat producers to being energy producers. And it was the extra air—not the exercise—that did it.

Energy production without oxygen is inefficient. Our cells *can* do it. It's called anaerobic metabolism. But aerobic metabolism is sixteen times better at producing energy. That's why aerobic exercise launched the fitness revolution.

This is probably a good time to mention that I have nothing against exercise. In fact, I'd have to call myself an enthusiastic proponent of the stuff. By all means, exercise every chance you get. All I'm saying is that if you can't exercise—because of time constraints, too much weight, or whatever—you can still pump your body with oxygen by practicing better breathing.

TAKE A BREATHER

VITAMIN O

"LACK OF OXYGEN IN THE TISSUES IS THE FUNDAMENTAL CAUSE FOR ALL DEGENERATIVE DISEASE."
STEPHEN LEVINE, PH.D.,
MOLECULAR BIOLOGIST

Oxygen is something we take for granted. We don't have to pay for it. We can't even see it.

Lately, however, oxygen has come into vogue. In Canada, bars serve "shots" of pure oxygen. In Japan, people pay big bucks to hang out in oxygen booths. And, of course, who can forget Michael Jackson's hyperbaric oxygen chamber.

Fad or not, no one can dispute that oxygen is a vital element in good health. In 1931, Dr. Otto

Warburg, a Nobel Prize—winning German doctor, discovered that normal, healthy cells turn malignant when they don't get enough oxygen.

Oxygen, we now know, plays a critical role in the proper functioning of the immune system. Because of its ability to kill infections, bacteria, viruses and other parasites, oxygen has been used to treat salmonella, cholera, and E. coli. One doctor even uses stabilized oxygen to purify water in Third World countries.

Many companies have sprung up in the last few years offering oxygen "pills." A quick scan of the Internet will show hundreds of companies that sell allotropic oxygen. Believers claim the following benefits:

- Boosts energy levels
- Strengthens the immune system
- Heightens concentration and alertness
- Calms the nervous system
- Kills infectious bacteria
- Enhances the uptake of vitamins, minerals, amino acids, and other essential nutrients
- Eliminates built-up toxins and poisons in the cells, tissues, and bloodstream

Let me tell you a story about a woman I know. Her name is Sondra Ray and if anybody breathes fully it's Sondra.

She's written two or three books on breathing. She's made an entire career out of what she calls rebirthing—a method of breathing where you connect your inhale and your exhale. And, yes, she's skinny. She could probably stand under a clothesline during a rainstorm and not get wet.

I met Sondra four or five years ago in Cape Cod. At the time, Sondra wasn't exercising. Hadn't exercised in years. Probably still doesn't if I know her. Somebody at the seminar we were attending was chiding her for this inexcusable lapse in lifestyle.

"How can you expect to keep up with us fit people if you don't exercise?" was basically the sentiment floating around.

Sondra, in all her breathing confidence, came up with this challenge. "You find the most difficult aerobic class and I'll come do it with you." To make a long story short, Sondra not only kept up with all her challengers but she walked out of the class without so much as breathing hard. Everybody else was lying on the floor panting, totally spent.

Or consider this story about two brothers. One was a professional mountain climber; the other, an engineer. The engineer brother, however, happened to be a yoga fanatic, which is to say he practiced breathing. To do yoga without superior breathing is a little like playing baseball without a bat. Anyway, the two brothers decided to take some big mountain trek together. The yoga brother was fretting he'd never keep up. Since the conclusion to this story is pretty obvious (he kept up with the greatest of ease), I won't even waste your time.

Let's just say that breathing, like exercise, is highly effective at pumping up your oxygen. Which, in the long run, is what's really going to take off all that extra weight.

The Role of Exercise

Ever since Jane Fonda put on a leotard, the party line has been that exercise melts off fat. It's part of our national psyche. But keep in mind that it takes ten miles of running to burn up the thousand calories you purchased in the McDonald's drive-through lane. Consider that you'll have to spend at least six hours running, cycling, and rowing to work it all off. Or let's say you jump rope for thirty minutes. You eagerly check the calorie expenditure in your handy-dandy calorie book. Lo and behold, you've only burned up two hundred extra calories. At best, you might be entitled to an extra dinner roll. Whoop-di-do.

Fortunately, scientists now have a better handle on how exercise works. Your body keeps burning calories as long as twenty-four hours after exercise. Even after you stop moving, your energy wheels keep right on spinning, keep right on producing heat. Consequently, a person who exercises regularly begins using the same amount of energy at rest that other people do while they're moving.

All that extra oxygen is altering your cellular chemistry. Your cells aren't the same once they get loaded down with extra oxygen. They've got to act differently. They've got to come up with a new strategy. So what do your cells do to handle the oxygen surplus from exercise? They kick into oxidation mode.

Oxidation, basically, is a fancy word for burn. The extra oxygen stokes your fat-burning fires. The more oxygen you put into a fire, the faster it burns. In other words, you've changed from a fat-storing machine to a fat-burning machine. Your metabolism has no choice but to kick in.

The other point that bears mentioning is that the oxygen you get with exercise is used to keep your muscles from building up lactic acid, which induces fatigue, cramps, and aches. Deep breathing, on the other hand, brings in more oxygen than you need, which gives you extra energy and extra fuel to burn fat.

If you're serious about changing your weight, it is absolutely imperative that you, like your cells, find a new strategy. You've got to find a way to change your body chemistry on a permanent basis. Diets alone won't do it. Yes, you can probably drop a pound or two—maybe even five. But within weeks after you resume normal eating mode, you'll be back on the phone moaning to somebody that you need to lose weight again.

The only way to permanently change your weight is to change your body's chemistry. Exercise will do it. There are probably hormones and chemicals that will do it. But the easiest way, the most convenient way, the cheapest way to permanently alter your body's chemistry is to fill it full of oxygen. I'm telling you, folks. Deep breathing is the answer.

By using the breathing exercises in this book, you can tune up your body within three weeks. You can literally revamp your entire cellular structure. You can pump up your metabolism so it never has a tendency to make fat again.

TAKE A BREATHER

THE DEAD TROUT LOOK AND OTHER BREATHING TIPS

1. Never strain. Breathing is a natural function of the body and it's supposed to be enjoyable.

2. Never force air into your lungs.

3. Keep your mind blank by concentrating on the breathing itself.

4. Keep your jaw relaxed. We experts call this the dead trout look. It may not be the best strategy for impressing a date, but it's ideal for drawing oxygen into the lower lobes of your lungs.

5. Mildly contract the abdomen at the end of the breathing to expel that last stale air.

7

YOUR METABOLISM IS NOT SET IN STONE

"BREATH IS ALIGNED TO BOTH BODY AND MIND AND IT ALONE CAN BRING THEM TOGETHER."

THICH NHAT HAHN,

Buddhist monk and creator of breathing tapes

Don't say it. Don't even think it.

If you've ever blamed your weight problem on having a slow metabolism, you're probably not going to like this chapter. That tired, worn-out excuse is about to be tossed out the proverbial window.

I'm not going to be totally ruthless. I readily admit that you, like everybody else, have a propensity for a certain metabolism. For example, if you're a woman your metabolism is probably a little slower than the average man's. If you're not a kid anymore, it's probably not as fast as it used to be (your metabolism starts to slow down when you're in your twenties). And if your parents, grandparents, and every known ancestor is overweight, you might just have a slower metabolism than Olive Oyl.

But if sex, age, and heredity are the bottom line, how can we account for Jessica Tandy, Walter Hudson, and Lynette Feinstein? The late Jessica Tandy, as you know, was slim and trim right up until her death at eighty-five. Walter Hudson was the guy (and remember, males supposedly have a metabolism 5 to 10 percent faster than women) who weighed fourteen hundred pounds when he took a big spill on his way to the bathroom from his bed, where he'd spent nearly twenty-seven years, clothed only in sheets. If you remember the national news story, you know that it took an entire team of emergency workers (many of whom were skinny women) four and a half hours to lift him back to his bed. Lynette Feinstein was the slimmest girl in my high school. She was valedictorian of thin. Her parents, however, were the fattest people in the auditorium when we walked across the graduation stage.

I'm trying to make the point that age, sex, and heredity are just a tiny piece of the metabolism puzzle. Literally, hundreds of factors affect your metabolism, which, by the way, is constantly changing, constantly reflecting the ingredients you've given it to work with.

Most of the factors that affect metabolism are controlled by you. In other words, having a slow metabolism is your choice. Dr. Robert Giller, an M.D. who wrote a book called *Maximum Metabolism,* said that of the factors affecting metabolism, there are more under our jurisdiction than those that aren't.

This is good news.

In fact, the sooner you get this through your noggin, the sooner we can all go out and celebrate.

The efficiency of your metabolic rate is under your control. Which means you *can* change your metabolism. You *can* change the rate at which your body burns food.

Remember your body is only as good as the ingredients you've given it to work with. And while there are plenty of books detailing the types of food you should eat (complete with recipes), the types of exercise you should do (complete with diagrams), and on and on, this book is concerned with only one ingredient—the amount of oxygen you give your body.

In fact, concentrating on anything else is drastically missing the point. Your breathing affects every last one of your bodily functions, but none more than your metabolism. Breathing and metabolism are inseparable. And oxygen is *the* key—will always be the key—that unlocks your metabolic rate.

In fact, if you walked into a lab and said, "Doc, my metabolism is slow. Can you give me a reading?" he'd hook you to a machine (after, of course, you've handed over several hundred-dollar bills) and he'd measure the amount of oxygen your body expends while making energy. For every 4.8 calories, the average person's body burns one liter of oxygen. In other words, your metabolism is nothing but a measure of how much oxygen you burn.

Doesn't it only make sense that the more oxygen you give your body to work with, the higher your metabolism rate is going to be?

If you've been on the diet path for some time, you've probably heard a term called "set point." It's a theory that explains why diets don't work. The theory is that once you lose weight and give up your diet, your body will automatically return to the weight where it feels most comfortable.

This theory is, for the most part, true. Diets are temporary fixes.

If you want to permanently change your weight, you have to permanently change the way your body works. Give it a new "set point."

I don't know about you, but if I had the choice of going on a diet with all its deprivation, guilt, and grapefruit or changing my body's chemistry so I didn't need to go on a diet, I'd pick the latter.

That's what this book is about—not about counting calories or fat grams or anything else. It's about transforming your body, about changing your chemistry. If you follow through with the breathing exercises in this book, you can completely revamp the chemistry of your body. By fully oxygenating your body, you can literally change your cellular structure at a very deep level. Which means you won't ever have to worry about fat grams at breakfast again.

Through breathing, you can turn your body from a sluggish, toxic landfill into a finely tuned, highly charged, metabolic masterpiece.

But first, let's take a look at what metabolism really is. When we talk about our metabolism, we usually talk about how fast we burn food. A person with a slow metabolism can limit his or her intake to carrots, peas, and tofu and will still gain weight. You've probably even said it yourself. "Everything I eat goes straight to my hips." Those lucky devils with the fast metabolisms can eat gallons of Ben and Jerry's "Cherry Garcia" and be hungry again in two hours. Their body just seems better able to process food.

Metabolism, if you ask a scientist, is the "sum total of all the chemical reactions that go on in living cells." It's the speed at which the body produces energy, not just energy for the digestion of Ben and Jerry's, but for all our bodies' numerous chores. Metabolism is the rate at which your body runs your brain, your heart, your liver, your kidneys, your fingernails, etc.

In fact, 75 percent of your body's energy is used for general maintenance. So a person with a higher metabolism will burn food faster and grow fingernails faster whether they're hiking up Mount Everest or playing tiddlywinks. This is your goal: to be an efficient fat burner at *all* times. In other words, you want to reconstruct your resting (or basal) metabolic rate.

Breathing is the key to warming and waking up your metabolism. When you breathe more oxygen into your body, several things happen to speed up your metabolism.

First, the heat in your body rises. If you've ever had a backyard barbecue, you understand the principle of heat and oxygen. What do you do if that darn charcoal won't turn red? You blow on it! Likewise, the logs in a fireplace won't produce heat without oxygen. The more oxygen, the hotter the coals. The more oxygen, the bigger the fires.

And while this might sound like a tip useful for Campfire Girls, it's also imperative information for anybody wanting to lose weight. Thin people, people with high metabolisms, have a much higher thermic rate. So to pump up your metabolism, you need to heat up your cells' burners by giving them more oxygen. By breathing deeply, you can literally reset your thermostat.

Over time, you can build up your body's thermostat so it will always be better at burning up fat—while sleeping, sitting, or climbing Mount Everest.

Producing heat is also very effective in changing your cellular makeup. Think of what a glassblower can do with a piece of glass tubing. When it's heated, a solid glass tube can be shaped into all sorts of cool flower vases, swans, and Snoopy dogs. Without the heat, the tube would shatter if you tried to make Snoopy.

As our cells become heated by breathing, they, too, become more pliable, less rigid. They begin to open up, creating more space for intercellular fluids to circulate. They become better at bringing in nutrients and carrying off toxins. Heat detoxifies the organs and tissues and revitalizes the entire system.

In fact, nothing can help your body more than cleansing out metabolic wastes. Every day your body burns through billions of cells. As many as 700 billion cells are replaced each day with new ones. The old cells, however, are toxic and must be removed from the system. This is no big problem for someone whose body is functioning properly, whose breathing is full and robust.

But if you're not getting enough oxygen, those old cells and other metabolic wastes may be loitering in your body, demanding large chunks of your energy. That's energy that could be used for processing food and taking off weight.

By breathing deeper, you promote proper circulation of the body fluids within the kidneys, stomach, liver, and intestines.

When you don't get enough oxygen (and remember 90 percent of us don't), your metabolism automatically slows down. Your cells can't burn up the fat as fast as you take it in. Consequently, your metabolism moves into conservation mode.

Scientists have identified two major metabolic pathways—the ergotropic mode (that's the work mode) and the trophotropic (that's the vacation mode). Let's put it this way. If you were a boss and you were hiring one of these two metabolic pathways, you'd definitely want to offer the ergotrop more money. Plus benefits. The ergotropic mode always gets the job done. It burns up fat. The trophotrop, on the other hand, is kinda lazy. It prefers to store fat. Its thinking is "Why should I carry this fat out of the body when I can just as easily stick it in a cell?" If there aren't enough cells, it will even make new ones to dump that fat in.

When you don't get enough oxygen, your body automatically hires the work-shirking metabolism. But when you breathe deeply, you get to welcome the hardworking metabolism to your team.

Unfortunately, people with slow metabolisms also suffer from sluggish blood flow. Like your great aunt Ethel, it can't get around like it used to. The Chinese refer to the blood as a sacred, restless, red dragon that must be continually fed. Deep breathing is the button that feeds the dragon and keeps the blood moving.

Another characteristic of people with slow metabolisms is that their lymphatic system doesn't function properly. And since the lymph system is best compared to a sewer or a dump truck, when it doesn't work properly, your body turns into New York City during the trash strike. The garbage builds up. And again, deep breathing is the button that stimulates the lymph system.

The other thing that flushes out your system is good old H_2O. And what is water but two parts hydrogen and one part . . . oxygen. When your body doesn't get enough oxygen, it can't create enough water and can't flush away the toxins. The solution once again is to give your body more oxygen. That way all those excess hydrogen molecules (which left to their own devices in your body turn into fat) can link up with the extra oxygen to cleanse your system.

And if all this wasn't enough, there's still the issue of stress. Being stressed out is one of the main hazards of metabolism. How many times have you started a diet and done pretty well until some stressful event occurs, something like the arrival of your summer electric bill, or the heel on your new $120 pair of shoes breaking off in the escalator? When the body is faced with a stress of any kind—be it a simple traffic jam or a boss that was Attila the Hun in a former life—it responds by dumping anti-stress (adrenal) hormones into the body. The most common is norepinephrine. This is a good thing except when your norepinephrine reserve is depleted, your body's metabolism screeches to a halt—or at least slows way down. What's worse, when the norepinephrine levels are low, insulin, the hunger hormone, pours in.

I know I'm starting to sound like a broken record, but deep breathing is also the best remedy for stress. If you don't believe me, ask the American Medical Association. The *Journal of the American Medical Association* has published numerous articles about using diaphragmatic breathing to eliminate stress.

Perhaps deep breathing sounds too good to be true. Could it really be the answer to all these problems?

The answer is yes. By learning to breathe properly, by fully oxygenating your cells, you can reset your metabolism to a much higher level.

TAKE A BREATHER

FREE BREATHING

"THE TRUE MAN BREATHES WITH HIS HEELS."
CHUANG TZU,
TAOIST PHILOSOPHER

HERE are some of the characteristics you'll find when you're really breathing freely.

- Your whole body moves in waves. For a good role model, watch a sleeping baby.
- Your rib cage is flexible and expands like elastic.
- The central diaphragm does the majority of the work.
- The breath expands in all directions, radiating out like a flower.
- There's a feeling of calm in the body and mind.
- It's effortless.

8

THE SOMEWHAT DRY BUT MANDATORY CHAPTER ON HOW YOUR BODY WORKS

"IN MY MEDICAL OFFICE, I RECOMMEND DEEP BREATHING TO ALL MY PATIENTS. I WRITE A PRESCRIPTION TO 'TAKE TWO BREATHS BEFORE MEALS AND AT BEDTIME AND AS NEEDED.'"

RONALD W. DUSKIN, M.D.

I'm not going to bore you with an entire college text on human respiration. Believe me, I've read dozens of them and they're not pretty.

But there are a couple of things you should know.

For starters, you should understand that your body is made up of some 75 trillion cells. And that the health of your body is entirely dependent on the health of those cells. If your cells are lean, mean, fighting machines, then guess what? You're a lean, mean, fighting machine. If, on the other hand, your cells are polluted and weighed down with all kinds of toxins, then they're going to be tired and so are you.

In fact, nothing can better predict your sense of well-being, your level of energy, and even your weight than those teeny, tiny cells that you can't even see without a microscope.

The reason those cells are so all important is because they produce the energy that runs your body. Each one of them, in fact, is a full-time chemical processing plant. While you're watching "Oprah" or playing the piano or even taking a catnap before dinner, those little dynamos are busy processing literally thousands of chemical reactions. They work twenty-four hours a day, seven days a week. They don't get weekends or vacations. They slave away night and day to turn these numerous chemical reactions into energy.

And while you may think this energy is used only for such physical outbursts as opening and closing your refrigerator door or chasing your toddler out of the pile of toilet paper he just unwound in the bathroom, the truth is that the energy your cells produce is also used for operating your kidneys, growing your hair, and sloughing off dead skin on your elbows. In fact, 75 percent of the work your cells do has nothing to do with physical activity. It has to do with simply maintaining your body.

As you can see, your cells have a pretty heavy load to carry. They have full-time responsibility for doing all the millions of things that bodies do—patching up bloodied knees, turning carbohydrates into glucose, moving blood from Point A to Point B.

Needless to say, all of these millions of nonstop activities require fuel—lots and lots of it.

This is where respiration comes in. The fuel that runs your body is oxygen. Granted, your body requires food and water, too, but the key ingredient that turns that food and water into energy is none other than simple, everyday oxygen.

Unfortunately, most of us aren't getting *enough* oxygen every day. So consequently, we're not providing our cells with the proper fuel.

While the body is great at storing reserves of carbohydrates, protein, and other necessities, it is impossible to store up oxygen. You must continue to supply it breath after breath.

I learned about oxygen the hard way. I'm one of these people who loves fires—campfires, fireplaces, candles by the bedside, you name it.

Despite my pyromaniac passion, I wasn't always so adept at starting fires. I'd stack pieces of wood up tightly, like Lincoln logs. I'd stuff newspaper under them, ignite my match, and watch, helplessly, while my fires—time and time again—sputtered and went out. Finally, some Colorado park ranger took pity on me and explained the importance of leaving space between the logs. They can't burn without oxygen, he pointed out.

Likewise, your cells can't operate without oxygen. They just won't work properly. You can eat sprouts for breakfast, tofu for lunch, and blue-green algae for dinner, but if you're not nourishing your cells with enough oxygen, they're never going to be completely healthy.

Back to the college text . . .

Your lungs, as I'm sure your seventh-grade biology teacher told you, are the tanks that hold the oxygen. Granted, it doesn't stay there very long. As soon as you inhale, these tiny balloon-like sacs that look an awful lot like a bunch of grapes (they're called alveoli, if you must know) filter oxygen into your bloodstream. At the same time that they dump oxygen into the blood, the grapes suck carbon dioxide out of your blood and send it back through your lungs into the atmosphere.

I like to think of the whole respiration process as a very organized waiter who brings you the menu, takes it away when you've decided what you want, brings you the food you ordered, and then clears away the plates when you've finished.

Now that you're fully trained in human respiration, let's talk about what happens when this intricately designed system runs amuck.

The blood taxi, a muscle which is better known as the heart, is surprisingly dependable at delivering blood to the cells. It doesn't waver much in most people.

Unfortunately, the same can't be said for the lungs. The amount of air we take in varies tremendously among people. Singers and athletes, for example, might take in seventeen pints of air with every breath. While others of us might breathe in less than two or three pints. Believe it or not, most of us take in less than one fifth of the oxygen our bodies need. That's 20 percent of what our lungs are capable of taking in.

TAKE A BREATHER

SHOW AND TELL

LET'S stop right now for a little "show and tell" break. See that body? Take out a marker and draw a diagram of the lungs. Don't worry about

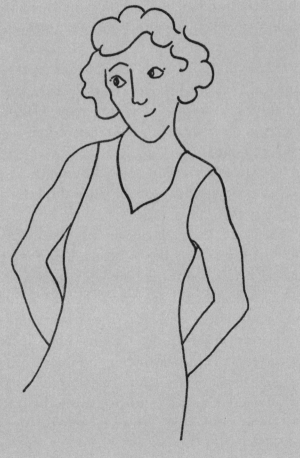

your artistic ability. Just draw in your best rendition of lungs.

Okay, now take a look at those lungs. How far do your penciled-in lungs extend? That's what I was afraid of. You drew them to start somewhere high on your chest and to stop right under the breasts.

This is a common misperception. Your lungs extend all the way down to your navel. In fact, they are shaped like a pyramid, so when you only breathe into the top part of your lungs (which is what most of us do), no oxygen reaches the important bottom portion. At the top of our lungs, the blood flow in the capillaries of the lungs is only a half teacup or so. At the bottom, the blood flow increases to ten times that much. Let's get the oxygen down to where it can be used.

So, in other words, your precious cells aren't getting enough fuel. They're literally being strangled, gasping for breath. If you've ever climbed to the top of a tall mountain, you know what I'm talking about. You can barely breathe, let alone carry on a conversation because your body isn't getting enough oxygen. That's how your cells are forced to operate pretty much every day. If they could talk, they'd be screaming "H-E-L-P."

Look at it like this. If you were getting only one out of every five hours of sleep you needed, you probably wouldn't feel very good nor would you be working at maximum capacity.

Likewise, your cells aren't feeling very good. Here they've got all these important responsibilities and they can't even get enough fuel to operate at maximum efficiency. They're operating on one of six cogs at best. It's like running a million-dollar Indy car on cheap gas. You were given a miraculous body. What a pity to feed it inferior fuel.

When our cells don't get the oxygen they need, several disastrous things happen.

Perhaps the worst is they get loaded down with toxins. They get gunked up with all sorts of awful things that not only slow down digestion but can eventually cause cancer, heart disease, and other things I'm sure you'd rather not talk about.

Wastes such as carbon dioxide and even dead cells must be moved out of the body. And since 70 percent of all wastes are processed through the breath (as opposed to the bowels and bladder), lack of oxygen causes wastes to accumulate.

This buildup of toxic wastes translates as fat. If you build up more toxic waste than you eliminate, it's got to be stored somewhere. Your body, in all its miraculous wisdom, refuses to store it in or near vital organs—at least for as long as possible. So where does it go? You guessed it: straight to your thighs, your buns, your waist, your upper arms, and fatty tissues in other parts of your body.

If the problem goes unchecked, the ultimate result is not only obesity, but general discomfort and life-threatening lethargy as the body spends all its energy on getting rid of the toxic wastes. No wonder you're too tired to jump on that StairMaster or for that matter get up and change the channel on the TV. Thank goodness for remote controls.

As it is now, with all these toxins, it's like stepping over a giant elephant every time you walk into the bathroom. You're not going to get there as fast as you could if the elephant were back in India or Africa where it belongs.

Adding to the problem, your blood chemistry gets screwed up. Because toxins are acidic, your acid-alkaline seesaw tips toward acid, which causes your system to retain water. After all, the extra water will help neutralize the acid. This, of course, adds even more weight, more bloat. Which causes you to breathe even higher in the chest, getting even less oxygen. The cycle is self-perpetuating. Once you rid your body of all the toxins, it can go to work processing the food you give it.

The other tragedy that occurs when your cells don't get enough oxygen is they convert from the fat-burning equilibrium to the fat-storing equilibrium. And while that's hardly good news for someone wanting to shed pounds, it's actually a tribute to your miraculous body.

In a nutshell, your cells are very advanced time management specialists. They know how to do the very best with what they've got. When they're not getting enough oxygen, it's only smart on their part to change from a metabolism that burns fat to a metabolism that doesn't. You see, it takes a lot of oxygen to burn up fat. And if your body isn't getting enough oxygen, it's only sound reasoning to form a fat cell because, well, it conserves the oxygen that's there.

If your circulation isn't delivering enough oxygen to

the cells, the fat-burning mechanism, like my tightly stacked logs, sputters and dies. Or at least kicks into energy-saving mode.

Now that you understand how your body works, you can see the importance of learning to breathe properly. If you were already breathing at maximum level, maybe then you'd have reason to throw your arms in the air. But since you're probably only breathing at one-fifth of your capacity, there is great hope.

All you have to do to clean out your system and lose weight is take in more oxygen through better breathing. Stick with this book and you'll learn how to increase your breathing—not just when you're doing the exercises—but at all times. Because once you retrain your body to breathe properly, it will work for you twenty-four hours a day.

It's as simple as this: If you start taking in more oxygen, your weight problem will take care of itself.

TAKE A BREATHER

THE MOST IMPORTANT MUSCLE IN THE BODY

SOME might argue that the brain is the most important muscle in the body, but without the diaphragm to supply it with oxygen, the brain is toast. In fact, the ancient Greeks used the word "diaphragm" for both the mind and the muscle that we call the diaphragm. This all-important dome-shaped muscle between the stomach and the chest automatically moves downward to draw air into the lungs and then moves up to press air out. The diaphragm is an invaluable tool. Once you understand how it works, try to "feel" the diaphragm in your own body.

THE WHOLE EARTH THEORY
OF WEIGHT LOSS

"HE LIVES AT A LITTLE DISTANCE
FROM HIS BODY."

JAMES JOYCE

Before we go any further, there's somebody you really need to meet. This is someone you should have met ages ago, someone who is and always has been your fiercest ally. Someone with all the answers. This modest know-it-all can award you the prize that has eluded you in the past.

Meet your body.

The main problem with your past efforts to lose weight is you've been looking in the wrong place. You've been searching for answers outside yourself. You've turned to Richard Simmons, Denise Austin, and doctors in white lab coats. You've conned yourself into believing that somehow they knew more than you, that they had more wisdom than your very own body.

It's like wanting to work on your relationship with your husband and then going to your aunt Ethel to talk about it. What in the world does your aunt Ethel know? She may be wise, she may have been married to your uncle Ernie for ninety years, and she may even have an advanced degree in marriage counseling, but she will *never* be able to do for you what a good talk with your own husband is going to do. You've got to go straight to the source.

In this case, the source of your difficulty is your body.

Through proper breathing, you learn to tune into your body. Breathing builds a bridge between your mind and your body. The two must become one.

Most dieters wage all-out war on their bodies, despising them because they refuse to stay in line. Consequently, there's no harmony, no union—just this angry, never-ending tug-of-war. We blame our bodies for everything. We look in the mirror and feel sick, desperately wanting to trade them in for a different model. Consequently, we become cut off from our bodies. It's us against them. No wonder we can't lose weight.

Maybe it's time to call a truce. Maybe it's time to do something radical, something like giving your body a little credit. Maybe, instead of constantly fighting it, you should actually sit down and invite it in for coffee. At least consider the possibility that it might, just might, know what it's doing.

Your body, that thing you've been referring to as a tub of lard, is actually a miracle of the finest dimension.

It's unmatched in intelligence, power, and flexibility. Those "love handles" that you detest are a sign of your body's great wisdom. Rather than dump excess fat in your heart or your kidneys, which might have polished you off by now, your very astute body dropped it off in a relatively benign spot. For now anyway, you can live with "love handles."

Your body's wisdom is staggering. It has five hundred muscles, two hundred bones, seven miles of nerve fibers, and enough atomic energy to destroy the entire city of Paris.

You just wouldn't believe all the astounding things that go on inside your body. Each day, your heart pumps blood over ninety-six thousand miles of blood vessels. That's like racing back and forth between Los Angeles and New York thirty-two times a day. Your eyes have 100 million receptors to take in sunsets and stars and the first smile of your grandbaby. Each of your ears has twenty-four thousand tissues to hear waves crashing against the shore, leaves rustling in the wind, Luciano Pavarotti singing an aria from *La Boheme*.

Each one of your cells performs more chemical reactions than all the world's chemical manufacturing plants combined. Your brain alone has 25 billion cells. That's more than six times the number of people on this planet. Each one of these little dynamos works with pinpoint precision without, I might add, any prompting from you. They didn't have to read a book or consult with Richard Simmons.

It is inconceivable that a masterpiece of this proportion would be left without the means to achieve a proper body weight. Did you get that? You might want to read that last sentence again. Your body has all the tools, all the instructions, all the blueprints you will ever need to achieve a proper body weight. Just as surely as you can see, hear, taste, and smell, you have the capability within yourself to be thin.

Granted, your body's thin may not be the same as Kate Moss's thin. But look inside and there's a body that's healthy, attractive, and if not Kate Mossian, at least thinner than the body you're hiding in now.

This may come as a surprise to you, but your body constantly strives to be fit. It's totally self-cleansing, self-healing, and self-maintaining. It doesn't really require a lot of help from you. Think about when you fall and skin your knee. Your body immediately forms a scab. Before you know it, that gash is healed, your knee is back to normal. Did you have to tell your body to do that? Did you have to run to the bookstore and buy an instruction manual on how to form scabs?

A robin doesn't need an architectural rendering to make his nest. Likewise your body knows what to do.

Face it, folks. Your pea-brain schemes are never going to cut it. You might as well surrender to the wisdom of your body.

You've got to learn to trust your body.

"But how?" you're probably protesting. "It's not like my body sends smoke signals."

Ah, but it does. Any time you get sick or gain a few pounds you have somehow defied your body's wisdom.

As you learn to breathe more fully, you can't help but get to know your body, you can't avoid hearing what your body is telling you. Breathing is the bridge.

You'll know when your body is really hungry. You'll

probably even know what it wants to eat. You'll begin to appreciate your body, honor it in all its magnificence.

For now, since we are somewhat cut off from our bodies, let's just look at the basics. And let's start with the lungs. Your lungs are capable of holding up to seventeen pints of air per breath. When you breathe in only two or three pints—which is the average for the adult American—you interfere with the magnificent tool your body has handed you. Why can your lungs hold seventeen pints of air? Just for kicks? I doubt seriously your lungs are there to take up space. They're capable of taking in seventeen pints of oxygen because that's how they work best.

When you get a beach ball, you don't fill it up one twelfth of the way and expect it to bounce properly. What fun are you going to have at the beach with a less-than-half-filled beach ball? We spend more time making sure our tires have enough air than our own bodies.

The thing that's different about this book is I'm not going to give you a formula for losing weight. How would I know what special formula would work for you? But I can give you the map that will help you access the inner wisdom of your body. As you begin to breathe, you'll start listening to your body. Breathing will help you to trust your body. Breathing will give you the answers. I don't know the answers. Nor does anyone else.

But the good news is your body does.

TAKE A BREATHER

PLACIDO DOMINGO, YOU'RE NOT

BUT singing—even singing badly—is a great diaphragmatic breathing exercise. Sing along with the radio every chance you get. This automatically exercises your abdomen and diaphragm. Your lungs will appreciate it even if your neighbors don't. Singing has actually been prescribed as a successful treatment for patients with blocked respiratory airways.

The best songs to sing are those with lots of words. The more words you have to squeeze in between breaths, the more you'll exercise your lungs and respiratory muscles. If you don't know the words, don't worry. You can still get all the benefits by singing "la, la, la" in time with the music.

1 0

OXYGEN: THE WONDER

DRUG

"INSUFFICIENT OXYGEN MEANS

INSUFFICIENT ENERGY."

NORMAN MCVEA, M.D.

The problem with diet pills and other pound-peeling medications is the side effects. I remember once, while taking Dexatrim, I was playing soccer on a Saturday afternoon. This wasn't just a group of friends playing a casual game. This was the Kansas City Swoop Park Women's B League Championship. I was playing halfback, a position where you can't really afford to lollygag around.

Midway through the second half, with the score tied three to three, this overwhelming pain shot through my side and I had no choice but to hobble off the field, clutching at my gut. I realized the week-long fix of Dexatrim was literally moving my insides to the outside. There's no getting around it. Drugs have harmful side effects. You can't put anything into the body (not water, not fiber, not anything) without your body making the proper corrections.

Oxygen, too, has side effects—things like glowing

skin, mental clarity, increased athletic performance (maybe if I'd been breathing instead of downing Dexatrim on a daily basis, our team wouldn't have lost the soccer championship, four to three), and, of course, spiritual enlightenment.

In fact, many doctors—including Harvard-trained Andrew Weil—believe breathing will play a predominant role in the art of human healing in the twenty-first century.

But for now, let's go over the benefits already discovered in this century. If you're one of these Doubting Thomas types, you may want to skip this chapter. If you're having a hard enough time swallowing that breathing will strip off extra pounds, you may want to wait and discover these pleasant offshoots for yourself.

INCREASED ENERGY. Let's start with the biggie. Deep breathing gives you so much more physical energy that you won't be able to sit around and moan about your tight clothes, your low metabolism, your . . . (fill in your excuse of choice). When you start breathing properly, you'll have so much more energy that you'll feel like dancing, maybe even starting that painting project you've been putting off. Who knows, maybe you'll ride a mountain bike over Pikes Peak. Whatever those long-lost goals, you'll suddenly find the energy and stamina to complete them. You'll find yourself springing out of the bed in the morning, excited about life.

When your cells don't get enough oxygen, they don't have the fuel to slough off toxins. And since this is one of their major jobs, they get bogged down and tired. They inefficiently spin their wheels, using what little fuel *is* available to keep trying. That's one thing you can say about your cells—they certainly don't give up easily. It's just that without the proper oxygen, their efforts to get rid of cellular pollution are futile. They're in a perpetual state of distress, which perpetually sucks your energy. Remember, you are only as healthy as your cells.

The good news is that by simply supplying them with an ample supply of oxygen, their job of removing toxic wastes is a piece of cake. And there's plenty of energy left over for you.

The other thing you'll notice when you start breathing properly is your energy level will be more consistent. You won't have those bursts of energy in the morning and then feel like sneaking into the bathroom for a snooze after lunch. Your energy will remain steady.

MIND-BODY HARMONY. If nothing else, breathing promotes mindfulness. It forces you to stay in the present moment. It's pretty hard to think about what to wear next year to the company Christmas party when you're shooting great wafts of air into your lungs. Oftentimes, the simple act of paying attention is the button that activates your healing.

The other advantage to uniting your brain and your body is that when they work together as a team, miracles can happen. If you've been on the diet path for any time at all, you've certainly run across one of the many books on thinking yourself thin. These books stress the importance of your mental disposition. If your brain is constantly putting yourself down and calling you "a loser," how can your body really do anything productive?

It's a constant tug of war. It's why people who faithfully do affirmations and picture themselves looking like Rene Russo end up looking more like a fullback for the San Francisco 49ers. Something is blocking the mind-body bridge—something like their subconscious, which believes they don't deserve to be thin or that they're really a fat pig and always will be. The good news is breathing can loosen that stuck lever—get the connection going again.

REDUCED STRESS. In this society of daytimers, honking traffic, and superman expectations, anything that curtails stress is worth checking out. Even choosing which of 120 television channels to watch can be a frenetic experience.

The good thing about slow, deep breathing is it will calm your mind, rein in all those whirling dervish worries that have taken off in seventy-eight different directions. Anytime you're feeling anxious or worried, let's say your teenager just got his driver's license, all you need do is stop for a minute, take a few deep breaths down in your belly, and *voilà!* the stress—if not gone—is at least manageable. Tension has melted from your body.

Cutting stress is particularly helpful if you're one of those people who consumes mass quantities of Baskin-Robbins when you're stressed out. Breathing will help you remain calm whereas Baskin-Robbins will only temporarily medicate. Being calm and living in a relaxed state also does wonders for your circulatory system, not to mention your metabolism. You'll be much better at digesting food if you're walking around with the demeanor of Mother Teresa instead of that of the Tasmanian Devil.

MENTAL CLARITY. The brain is oxygen's best customer. It takes a lot of juice to run that intricate mass of tissue in your skull. In fact, the brain, which is less than 3 percent of your body's weight, uses 20 percent of your body's oxygen.

When it's flooded with oxygen, it just plain and simple works better. Although I've never seen a study on this, I'd be willing to wager that Einstein and Thomas Edison and all those other genius types were healthy breathers.

Deep breathing helps you concentrate better, solve problems more easily, and probably even balance your checkbook faster. Deep breathing is a must on the job— especially in the afternoon when post-lunchtime lethargy sets in. Taking a deep breath will revive you and it will also make your boss wonder what you're up to.

And when it comes to weight loss, the advantages to mental clarity are obvious. I mean how smart is it to eat two banana cream pies at one sitting? If your brain is functioning like a well-oiled top, you'll be so busy solving world problems that overeating won't even be a consideration.

SELF-ESTEEM. Is the motto "life sucks" your calling card? Do you wake up in the morning thinking "Well, only sixteen hours until I can go to bed again"? If so, you need to take a deep breath right this very minute.

From a purely scientific standpoint, breathing helps

your mood because it pumps endorphins into your system. Endorphins are natural feel-good chemicals. They can even serve to mask pain. It's how rock climbers with cuts on their hands can keep going. Their body is so pumped with endorphins they don't even notice that their right knee is bleeding and their left thumb is about to fall off. It's also why Lamaze classes teach pregnant mothers how to breathe. I even heard a story once about a guy who breathed his way through dental visits without using anesthesia. This, in my opinion, is carrying the oxygen thing a little too far.

ATHLETIC PERFORMANCE. Nowadays, there aren't many Olympic caliber athletes who don't pay attention to their breathing. It's just too important. Gay Hendricks tells the story of a marathon runner who dropped thirty minutes from her marathon time after just one breathing lesson. Dr. James Loehr, a contributing editor to *Tennis* magazine, writes articles on the benefits of using oxygen to jazz up your tennis game. It may sound like Monica Seles is grunting when she's firing off a serve, but she's actually focusing her breath (and her energy) for ultimate power.

The reason Jackie Chan and other martial arts bigwigs say "aa-ya" when they break boards is because that forceful noise directs the breath and the energy.

Sports Illustrated even reported a story about a seventh-grade softball team from Mesa, Arizona, that went from last place to first when they began doing breathing exercises before each game.

When you breathe deeply through your nose, your muscles relax, your blood pressure falls, your nerves are calmed, and consequently you have more endurance, more focus, and fewer injuries. John Douillard, owner of LifeSpa in Boulder, Colorado, has taught everyone from former Secretary of the Treasury Bill Simon to Billie Jean King to find "the zone" in their fitness program by breathing deeply through the nose.

In order to improve your serve or your golf swing or your time in a three-legged race, you should focus on lengthening the breath and coordinating it with the natural rhythms of your arms and legs. It will help your sport more than the best pair of shoes.

TAKE A BREATHER

WORLD-CLASS BREATHERS

"FOR ATHLETES, OXYGEN IS THE MOST IMPORTANT FUEL."

BARON BAPTISTE, YOGA TEACHER

THIS is just a partial list of athletes who have studied breathing.

- Martina Navratilova
- Stan Szozda, Polish world champion bicyclist
- Herschel Walker
- Kareem Abdul-Jabbar
- The entire Philadelphia Eagles football team

- Billie Jean King
- Alexi Grewal, '84 Olympic gold medalist in bicycling
- Jackie Joyner-Kersee
- Danny Manning
- All participants in the Carpenter/Phinney Bike Camps

BETTER SEX. (OR, THE SECTION YOUR MOTHER SHOULDN'T READ.) Speaking of athletic performance: There are many reasons your sex life will soar when you begin to practice better breathing. All of the above play a significant part: the energy, the lack of stress, the self-esteem.

But most important, as you really allow yourself to get in touch with your body, you'll feel things you've never felt before. Every breath will trigger pleasant sensations. Gay Hendricks once asked a room of advanced breathwork students how many had noticed an improvement in their sex lives. Nearly all of them raised their hands. Breathing right enhances the body's ability to feel positive energy. You're liable to become so orgasmic you won't know what to do. Come to think of it, maybe we'd better keep this one between ourselves.

DEWY, FRESH SKIN. When you start breathing better, one of the first things you'll notice is the change in your skin tone. Gay Hendricks says that invariably his therapy clients started looking younger. Sure, they were there to work on their relationship with their husband or to get over their fear of heights. But once they started breathing properly (the first thing he has every client do), their skin really perked up.

What you may not realize is that the skin, your body's largest organ, is one of the key players in the toxic elimination department. When the breathing mechanism falls down on the job, the skin is forced to take on double duty. Without adequate oxygen, you're liable to wake up one day, look in the mirror, and see Georgia O'Keeffe staring back at you.

As you discover the full potential of your lungs, your skin will celebrate its newfound freedom by looking good.

My friends were amazed when I first started doing breathing exercises. They wanted to know what new makeup I had discovered.

VIBRANT HEALTH. Sheldon Saul Hendler, a doctor in San Diego who wrote a book called *The Oxygen Breakthrough,* believes futile breathing is the cause of a majority of our illnesses and says that "there is a bad breathing epidemic at large" today.

In fact, he says breathing is the first place, not the last, one should look when fatigue, disease, or other evidence of disordered energy presents itself.

He contends that the underlying factor in all infection, allergies, hormonal disturbances, nutritional deficiencies, and on and on is what he calls "oxygen interruption." By teaching his patients better breathing techniques, he's been able to "cure" them of everything from allergies and arthritis to fibrositis and chronic fatigue. He also says that a significant number of people who think they have heart disease are actually suffering from breathing disorders. One study showed all 153 patients of a coronary unit breathed predominantly into their chests.

The heart disease contention was borne out by a Dutch study that compared two groups of heart attack patients. Group A was taught simple, diaphragmatic breathing, while Group B was left to their own breathing devices. Over the next two years, seven of the twelve patients in Group B had second heart attacks while none of the subjects in Group A had further attacks.

Another medical researcher estimates that poor breathing plays a role in more than 75 percent of the ills people bring to their doctors. In most cases, poor diaphragmatic breathing is the culprit.

I've had many clients overcome illnesses. Scott, a thirty-eight-year-old salesman, had suffered from irritable bowel syndrome for years. His doctors chalked it up to his high-stress job. When he started doing breathing exercises, he not only dropped twenty pounds in a short two months, but his IBS disappeared completely. Even though he's on the road constantly and can't find time to exercise, he doesn't go a day without one hundred deep belly breaths.

Nobel Prize winner Dr. Otto Warburg said that cancer has only one cause—the replacement of normal oxygen respiration by oxygen-deficient respiration.

So while you may be reading this book because you want to be slim and trim, the real reason may be to overcome a chronic illness. Many people who begin breathing exercises wind up with what they consider to be a miraculous physical healing.

It's actually anything but miraculous. If your breathing isn't operating at peak efficiency, your toxins aren't being released properly, which forces your kidneys and your heart and your other organs to work overtime. Needless to say, this sets the stage for any number of illnesses.

REDUCED HOT FLASHES. In a study reported in the *American Journal of Obstetrics and Gynecology,* deep breathing exercises helped menopausal women reduce their hot flashes by 50 percent.

Okay, I admit this all sounds too good to be true. Particularly when you figure you've been sitting on this secret for all of your adult life.

I like to think of that classic story called *Acres of Diamonds*. A man named Ali Hafed dedicated his life to finding the planet's biggest diamonds. He sold his home, left everything he knew, and set out on a worldwide expedition to find diamonds. Finally after years and years of fruitless trying, Ali Hafed returned home, a spent and broken man. And guess what? The diamonds that had eluded him were right there in his own backyard.

TAKE A BREATHER

A BREATH OF FRESH AIR

THE quality of the air you breathe is important. Get outside at every opportunity. Think how wonderful it feels to breathe in air from a pine forest or from a salty ocean breeze.

Put plants and flowers in your house. Remember they put out oxygen.

Every day, even in sub-zero temperatures, air out your house for a few minutes. This means opening a couple of windows. The good news for those afraid of heating bills is fresh air heats a lot faster than recycled air.

PART TWO

THE
PROGRAM

"IF YOU GREET THE AIR WITH
GENTLENESS, IT WILL SHARE WITH
YOU THE MAGIC OF ITS POWER."

RUMI, PERSIAN POET (1207–1273)

THE ENERGY COCKTAILS

Breathing right is a lifetime commitment. It's definitely not a Band-Aid or a quick fix. It's my hope that you'll look forward to using this program for the rest of your life.

If you prove to your body that you're serious about listening to its wisdom, I guarantee you'll get the answers you're looking for. Albert Schweitzer dubbed it "giving the doctor who resides within the chance to go to work."

And all you have to do is show up.

Breathing will allow your body to heal itself, to right any imbalances. Trust this. Take it seriously.

Give this program the chance to sink in. Let yourself feel it deeply. Commit to doing it every day. After you've got the hang of it, it's fine to modify it for your own needs. Remember, this is *your* body you're listening to, not mine.

Honor each and every breath. The breath is so subtle, has so many avenues to lead you down that it's worth slowing down the journey.

But whatever you do, don't read through this section, think to yourself, "You know, that just might work," and then make a date to do them . . . later. Later never comes. Please don't fall into that trap.

The breath within you has the power to change your life. Give it the reverence and the respect it deserves.

The daily maintenance program includes three breathing exercises. I call them "energy cocktails." Do each one until you've made it "yours." After you've mastered these, experiment with the other cocktails.

Take your time. Savor each cocktail like a hot cinnamon bun straight from the oven.

Carola Speads, a breathing coach in New York City, insists that her students limit themselves to one new "breathing experiment," as she calls them, each week. Only when they've mastered one are they ready for the next.

There is also an "olive" at the end of each cocktail—some food for thought, some extra morsels that you may want to digest while you're breathing deeply.

It is my deepest hope that these exercises bless your life and lead you to the answers you've been searching for.

The Daily Menu

By now, you've undoubtedly mastered deep belly breathing. You're taking long, slow, deep breaths in the shower, while applying eyeliner, even between sneaking peaks at your horoscope in the magazines at the grocery checkout counter. You're especially remembering to stop and take a breath every time you feel panicky or stressed.

Your lungs, your ribs, and that ever-important diaphragm muscle are loosening up. In fact, you're feeling so much better, exploding with so much energy that you'd wish I'd just shut up and get on with it.

You win.

Here is the basic daily menu for turning your body into a finely tuned masterpiece.

1. DO THREE SETS OF TEN "BAYWATCH BI-KINI BREATHS" (SEE PAGE 119 FOR INSTRUC-TIONS). That's thirty total energy cocktails. Every day. It shouldn't take more than five or six minutes each time you do a set of ten. It's a good idea to begin your day with a set of ten. That way your metabolism is off to a roaring start. You'll feel so much better and have so much more energy that you won't mind getting up a few minutes earlier.

But if you should forget, don't beat yourself up. Just make sure you get them in before you go to bed. Remember, this plan is about ease, convenience, lowering stress.

After meals is also a good time to whip out a set of ten. If at all possible, stand up when you do them. If you can't (remember the point is to DO them), fit them in while sitting in your office, driving the kids to soccer, or drying the dishes. Whatever you do, do thirty every day.

2. TAKE TEN QUICK "KUNG FU BREATHS" BE-FORE EACH MEAL. The key to health and a thin body is a properly functioning digestive system. This simple breath only takes a few seconds, but it will stoke your digestive fires. Try to get in ten before every meal. If not ten, do five (see page 123 for instructions).

3. WALK AROUND THE BLOCK (OR FOR A MIN-IMUM OF FIVE MINUTES) ONCE A DAY WITH YOUR MOUTH FULL OF WATER. Sounds crazy, I

know, but this is what Apache warriors did when they were training for big showdowns. To build stamina and instill discipline, they would run across the desert with their mouths full of water. You're doing it to improve your breathing. If you don't want to use the water, just make sure to keep your mouth closed. For the entire walk, breathe only through your nose. If your aerobic capacity is really bleak, you may feel at first as if you're suffocating. Slow down if this should happen, but *do not* switch to mouth breathing.

Don't think of it as exercise. Think of it as a great way to pump your body with oxygen. It takes only five minutes and since you're going to have so much extra energy now that you're breathing properly, you're going to need somewhere to put it. Maybe you'll even feel like walking two or three blocks. One is all that's required. Five minutes is all that it takes.

Not only will you get several gallons of extra oxygen in your walk, but it will be fresh air—as in refreshing, invigorating, energizing.

Don't let things like rain, snow, and sleet prevent your one-block romp. If the postman can do it, you can, too. Remember there are things like raincoats, boots, and down-filled jackets.

Okay, that was the basic menu. What could be easier than this?

Add the following for dessert.

4. EACH WEEK, EXPERIMENT WITH A DIFFER-
ENT ENERGY COCKTAIL. You're already doing

thirty Baywatch Bikini Breaths, thirty Kung Fu Breaths, and walking one block—every day. There are eleven more energy cocktails to try in the pages that follow. Try to set aside fifteen minutes three or four times a week, for the next eleven weeks, to experiment with each of these energy cocktails. Stick with just one for the whole week. Get to know it. Find out what lessons it has to teach you, what benefits it offers to your life.

You'll be tempted to try a whole lot of the cocktails right away. Don't sabotage yourself. This "do it all" mentality is what gets us in trouble. Slow down.

Breathing is so deceptively simple that it often takes a while to master. Trust that. Some of the exercises you might not like, but don't toss them out the window just yet. It could be you're resisting that particular cocktail because it's just the one you need.

COCKTAIL ONE:
Baywatch Bikini Breath

This breath is the very best one I know for fully oxygenating your body, increasing your energy, and losing weight. If you do just this one breath, ten times, three times a day you will revolutionize your life. You'll lose weight, become a genius, and be writing books of your own.

Here's how it works:

1. Stand up and say, "I am the greatest"—not only out loud, but in your posture. Remember, your body speaks volumes.

2. Take a long slow belly breath, inhaling through your nose.

3. Lock the breath inside your body and hold it for four times as long as you inhaled. For example, if you inhaled to the count of four, hold it to the count of sixteen.

4. Now, exhale through your mouth twice as long as you inhaled. Again, using the four example, exhale to the count of eight.

The ratio is always one—four—two. If you breathe in to the count of five, it's hold for 20 (four times five), exhale for ten (two times five). If it's three, it's hold for twelve, exhale for six. You get the picture.

After a while, you'll notice that your lung capacity is improving. At first, your inhale might only last to three counts. Eventually, you'll be able to inhale to the count of eight or ten or who knows? Remember your lungs are muscles that get better with use.

The reason you hold the breath inside your body is because it floods your cells with health-giving energy. The extra-long exhale squeezes out toxins.

And if you're going to do something, you might as well make it fun. So I've come up with this modification.

Forget about numbers. After all, how much fun is it to count to seven over and over again. You simply inhale as long as it takes to mentally say, "Baywatch Bikini, here I come."

Then you hold the breath inside your body, "Baywatch Bikini, here I come once. Baywatch Bikini, here I come twice. Baywatch Bikini here I come thrice. Baywatch Bikini, here I am." Now you let it out or exhale to "Baywatch Bikini, here I come once. Baywatch Bikini, here I come twice."

And you do this ten times. Three times a day. If Baywatch Bikini gets old and tiresome, make up your own mantra. Something like "I am skinny, look at me." or "Eat your heart out, I'm a babe." Be creative. Have fun. Just make sure you inhale deeply for as long as you can. It's in through the nose, out through the mouth. Remember, never strain. Just make it a deep, relaxing, enjoyable breath.

This is the breath I learned from Tony Robbins. He claims that this one breath changed his life. Just remember to do it three times a day. It's particularly powerful to try it right after you eat. Your metabolism always kicks in after a meal because, well, it now has extra work to do. By giving it extra oxygen, your body's metabolism can work at warp speeds.

THE OLIVE:

Make Breathing Fun

''Breathing's a great way to get stoned without the side effects.''
TOM ROBBINS, AUTHOR OF
EVEN COWGIRLS GET THE BLUES

Diets are the enemy. They make you paranoid, insane, and fat. They are the main obstacle between you and your ideal weight.

I mean who wants to start anything that spells deprivation, starvation, and the end of all chocolate as we know it today. It's like inviting this nasty little gnome to sit on your shoulder, shake his crooked, gnarled finger at you, and say "naughty, naughty" every time you have a pleasant thought. Diets are unnatural.

It's no wonder you keep putting it off until next Monday or "Hey, it's Thursday now, I might as well pig out until next week when I can get serious" or "Well, there's just not enough ice cream to put back in the refrigerator. I might as well finish it up tonight. I can start tomorrow."

What I'd like to suggest is a weight-change strategy that's fun. Something you'd actually look forward to. Like meeting Richard Gere for cocktails or picking out which pair of Evan-Picone pumps you'd like for free.

Human beings are very crafty at avoiding pain. It's programmed in like the need to eat, sleep, and, when you're about to turn thirty-five, have babies. So the only hope of ever changing your weight permanently is to turn your strategy into something you simply can't wait to do. Like breathe! Why wait until tomorrow when you could start right now?

Quit taking your weight so darn seriously. Whether or not you fit into your size-six stretch pants is not going to alter the Middle East peace talks. At one point, I considered titling my book *Baywatch Bikini, Here I Come*, but I was advised that people who buy weight-loss books would never go for anything *fun*. Heaven forbid that we should enjoy ourselves. Losing weight is tough work and we've got to take it seriously. In my humble opinion, that's the crux of the problem.

Once we put our weight in perspective and realize we're going to die someday whether we weigh eighty pounds or eight hundred, it's a lot easier to laugh at ourselves.

Even the term "diet" (which I've already pointed out starts with the word "die") or the term "weight loss" prevents our accomplishment. Why do we have to lose anything? It's much preferable to think about gaining something—like health and beauty and a body like Raquel Welch.

COCKTAIL TWO: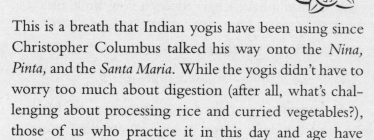

Kung Fu Breath

This is a breath that Indian yogis have been using since Christopher Columbus talked his way onto the *Nina, Pinta,* and the *Santa Maria.* While the yogis didn't have to worry too much about digestion (after all, what's challenging about processing rice and curried vegetables?), those of us who practice it in this day and age have discovered that it does wonders for the digestive system.

When we're not completely relaxed (say sixteen hours of the day) our belly muscles tighten, our breath shifts to our chest, and our involuntary nervous system kicks into overload. This neat impulse (often called the fight or flight response) prompts adrenaline to drip into our bloodstreams, our muscles to go on red-alert, and our digestion to slow down.

This breath will loosen up your belly, relax your muscles, and let your body digest its food more easily. It is particularly helpful to do five to ten of these before each meal. Think of it as setting the table. What this breath does is push air into what martial arts practitioners call the "hara." Since most modern medical diagrams don't list hara, let me tell you that it's an energy center located approximately two inches below your navel. The hara is used a lot in aikido, kung fu, and karate.

Here's how it works:

1. Stand up. Remember these exercises can always be modified to suit your needs. But whenever you can, stand up and act as if you mean it.

2. As you inhale deeply through your nose, tilt your head back as if you're looking to see if there's dust in the chandeliers.

3. Pause for just a millisecond before . . .

4. Exhaling forcefully through your mouth. Make a loud, definite "ha" sound as you bring your head back to its normal position.

At first it's a little embarrassing—especially if you're having brunch with your in-laws for the first time—but they'll get used to it. Maybe your in-laws will think you're training to be a samurai and will hold you in great esteem. At least they won't try to steal food off your plate.

And remember, if you ever feel bloated and are thinking R-O-L-A-I-D-S, think "K-U-N-G F-U" breath instead.

THE OLIVE:

Albert Einstein Theory of Weight Loss

"Directing the potency of your breath is like uncovering a Fort Knox of currency you never knew you had."
JEFFREY MIGDOW, M.D., CO-AUTHOR
OF *TAKE A DEEP BREATH*

I have a feeling that when Albert Einstein formulated the theory of relativity, he wasn't exactly thinking of its implications to the field of weight reduction. But then, I never met either of his wives.

However, Einstein's now-famous $E=mc^2$ has great relevance to you and your bathroom scales. Particularly as you learn to breathe more fully. Because the real purpose of breathing is not to move air, but to move energy.

The Chinese have known about this vital human energy for centuries. Long before there was an Albert Einstein or a United States of America, for that matter, the Chinese were working with their "*chi*." Translated into English that means "vital life force." To this day, the

Chinese believe that all illness is caused by some blockage in the *chi*. Millions of them (and I hasten to point out that you don't see many fat Chinese) arise at dawn morning after morning to practice "Qi Gong," a form of exercise that focuses on breathing. The Indian yogis had a different name for it (prana), but it's basically the same thing. Energy. And the key to harnessing it is your breath.

Energy is a pretty nebulous thing. You can't see it or take it out to dinner. But it's something we all recognize. Something we all talk about. "Man, do I ever have lots of energy today" or "Well, I'd love to type your 190-page term paper for you, but, well, I'm feeling low in energy."

When you learn to breathe fully (especially if you make it an important daily practice), you will become more aware of this energy. You'll be able to direct it, to steer it in ways that help you. As it is now, your energy is probably unfocused.

You have this incredibly powerful force and you're not using it. You're not capitalizing on this almighty life force that's certainly a lot bigger than your wimpy weight problem.

The other thing you should understand is that your body itself is energy. A lot of us believe our bodies are static matter, frozen statues. But physicists tell us it just ain't so.

In one of my first breathing trainings, I was supervising a woman who was learning to breathe differently. She had a blanket over her body and as I watched her breathing accelerate, I noticed these waves moving up and down the blanket. It looked like the Atlantic Ocean— not big enough waves to surf on, but definitely big enough to wash in a few clams. I assumed there was an air-conditioning vent blowing into the blanket, although I'd never seen a air conditioner make waves like that.

Much to my surprise (and believe me, I checked several times after that session was over), there was no vent, absolutely nothing that would have made those waves— except the energy pulsating through that woman's body.

Our bodies are rivers of energy—constantly changing, continuously flowing. If you could really "see" the atoms that make up your cells, you'd see them constantly be-bopping from one place to another. What we "see" with our eyes is more like the outline left by a Fourth of July sparkler—no longer there, but still visible.

In fact, your body is different now than it was when you started reading this chapter. Wait five days and every atom in your stomach will be different. Within six weeks, the atoms that make up your DNA will be entirely new. And after four years, every atom of your physical body will be completely replaced.

So breathe, breathe, breathe, and get that energy moving in the direction you want it to go.

COCKTAIL THREE:

Guided Tour

We've been talking about lungs, diaphragms, and other body parts that aren't normally tossed into everyday conversation. It's important as we become reacquainted with our bodies to "feel" our own body parts, to understand how our own personal breathing mechanism works. Let's just call the next three cocktails a crash course in "getting to know you."

I adapted the following one from Gay Hendricks's book, *Conscious Breathing*. According to Hendricks, it's important to take an internal guided tour of your body so you can have a conscious feeling-picture of how your breathing works and why it is designed the way it is. Use your consciousness as a searchlight.

Try doing this breath once a day. Let's get started:

1. Lie down. Rest your arms at your side and take a couple of deep breaths.

2. Run your fingers along your collarbone. Notice where it touches your shoulders and where it connects to your sternum. Ball your hands into a loose fist and tap along the collarbone and then pause for a few seconds and tune in to your collarbone. You might even ask it a question.

3. Now, let's get in touch with your sternum. Like a stair step, trace down the sternum with your fingertips. Feel where each rib joins the sternum. Notice that the farther down you go, the closer the ribs are together. Feel just beneath the sternum and find a tiny bone called xiphoid process. This is connected to your diaphragm, the most important muscle in

your body. Again, take your loose fist and retap the same route. Stop and tune it.

4. From your xiphoid, trace your rib cage as it continues down. Feel how far down it goes. Gently and rapidly tap the edge of your rib cage with your fingertips. Notice that the bottom of your ribs is all the way down by your waist. Many of us think our lungs are high in our chest, but your lungs follow the structure you just traced of your rib cage. Lungs are small at the top and very large at the bottom. That's why it's so important to breathe down in the belly where the body needs the oxygen.

5. Now rest your hands at your side again. Use your consciousness to take the same tour your hand just did. Sense how your collarbone connects to your sternum, how it continues down to the xiphoid process, and how your ribs extend down to your waist.

6. Take several deep breaths, feeling how your rib cage expands with each breath.

7. Now let's pay attention to the diaphragm. Notice that it's shaped like a dome. Breathe in, flatten it.

8. Tighten your stomach muscles. Feel what it's like to have your breathing restricted by tight stomach muscles.

9. Create the fight or flight reflex. Lift your head

off the floor, make tight fists, tense your buttocks. Hold this for a moment. Try to take a few deep breaths. See!

10. Now, take a very clear mental and kinesthetic snapshot of your body and what it's like to try and breathe under that amount of tension.

11. Now let all muscles relax, take a few deep breaths, feeling your body swell as you breathe in and flatten as you breathe out.

THE OLIVE:

Put a Lock on It

> "**Your body is simply a living expression of your point of view about the world.**"
> CARL FREDERICK, AUTHOR OF
> *PLAYING THE GAME THE NEW WAY*

1. "I have a slow metabolism."

2. "It's really hard for me to lose weight."

3. "I just look at a piece of chocolate cake and gain weight."

How many times have you said 1, 2, 3, or all of the above? How often do you look in the mirror and think, "Oh, yuck"?

Not only do behaviors like this make you feel like warmed over dog doo, but they prevent you from dropping weight. Every time you say or think anything (whether it's negative or positive), your body listens and acts accordingly. The cells of your body eavesdrop on every word you say. Anytime you talk about something or even think about something, your cells react. In other words, you are constantly practicing neurochemistry.

Neurophysiological research tells us that the nature of our thinking automatically determines the nature of our bodily activities. In other words, if you turn the same thoughts about your weight over and over in your mind, they get lodged in the muscles and glands of your body. So when you make comments about your jiggly forearms or the tire tube around your tum, you're actually stamping those comments into the tissues of your body.

Even people who have gained only a few pounds are not serving themselves by pointing it out. It is much smarter to proclaim thinness.

Our bodies, neurophysicists tell us, are merely a barometer of our own belief systems. It's actually our beliefs about ourselves—more than the banana cream pie we couldn't resist—that cause us to gain weight.

Dr. Thomas Hanna, a famous energy worker who studied with Moshe Feldenkrais and others, says that when you look at a person's body, you're actually observing the moving process of that person's "mind." He says it's impossible to "think" without moving. So your body, in essence, is basically a physical representation of your thoughts.

The spoken word, particularly, is very powerful. Listen to what you say. Do you constantly put yourself down? Do you complain about your weight out loud on a regular basis?

From now on, pay attention to what you say. Every time you make a disparaging comment, turn it around—if not out loud, then at least silently to yourself. For example, your best friend calls and without thinking you casually mention that "I ate a whole bag of buttered popcorn at the movie yesterday. I probably gained eighteen pounds." Cancel it by saying something like, "Well, I'm not sure. I spilled half of the bag when Antonio Banderas first took off his shirt and I actually think I look thinner." You don't have to be modest. It's okay to admit to people that your buns look good and that you think you're a knockout.

COCKTAIL FOUR:

Stretch Your Breath

Well, now that you know where your xiphoid process is, how about putting it back to work? This next cocktail is great at limbering up the oxygen passageways. Do this sequence once a day.

1. Stand with your feet eighteen to twenty inches apart.

2. Clasp your hands behind your back and extend your arms down toward your heels.

3. As you inhale through your nose, lift and open your chest and rest your chin on your chest.

4. Feel the front lungs and chest inflating.

5. Exhale through your nose and release your chin.

6. Return to the neutral standing position.

7. Repeat three times.

8. Now, clasp your left wrist with your right and extend your arms in front of your body.

9. As you inhale through your nose, round your back and bend your knees so that your whole body is curling forward.

10. Feel the back lungs inflating.

11. Exhale through your nose and release, coming back to the neutral standing position.

12. Repeat three times.

THE OLIVE:

Trash Your Bathroom Scales

> ''**One of the greatest deterrents to doing anything well is trying to do it well.**''
> TIMOTHY GALLWEY, AUTHOR OF
> *INNER TENNIS*

Are you a flab fanatic? Do you make sure every last bit of clothing is removed—including your pinkie ring—before you weigh yourself? Do you measure success in life by how "good" you were at your last meal?

It would be one thing if this fuss over flab were constructive, but, ironically, putting energy into weight only makes you fatter. Obsessing over what you're going to eat next or what you're never going to eat again is counter-productive. Extra vigilance, in this case, does not work. What you eat for dinner shouldn't be any more problematic than balancing your checkbook or scheduling a dentist appointment.

Plus if you're so preoccupied with your weight you're often distracted from solving other problems. You see everything in your life—your dead-end job, your dead-beat boyfriend, your dead sex life—as revolving around your bathroom scales. If only I were skinny, I'm sure I could get another job. If only I could lose ten pounds, then I know I'd feel good enough to finish that deck my wife keeps bugging me about. . . . If only, if only . . .

Weight becomes a lightning rod for all of life's dissatisfactions.

So the first rule in this program is to forget about your weight. It is now a non-issue. Do not get on your scales. Not even one last time to see what your starting weight is. Do not wonder how many calories are in that half serving of peach yogurt.

Do not think about anything at all having to do with your weight or food or fat grams.

I'll warn you right now. This is going to be extremely difficult at first. I recommend you go cold turkey, but if you must, give up the scales on a gradual basis. You're going to feel antsy, bored, maybe angry. You might even decide, "to hell with it" and get back on the scales. Right now you are so accustomed to strategizing about your weight that your life will feel empty when you give it up. People claim to be addicted to food, but what they're addicted to is all the time and energy they invest in thinking about food.

When you're perennially worrying about diet-related issues, you have a built-in excuse for why you don't really live life. I mean if you didn't have those fat grams to count or those sit-ups you didn't do to feel guilty about you might just have time to walk to the park, visit an old friend, or write a letter to your mother.

Every time the subject comes up—let's say you start wondering how many extra pounds that last bag of chips contributed to your physique and you'd really like to get out the scales and take just a quick peek—take three deep abdominal breaths instead. Put your hand on your abdomen and really push that inhale into your gut. Focus on your breathing. Notice how it feels.

At first, you're going to be breathing every five minutes. You'll be shocked at how often the subject comes creeping into your brain. You'll be appalled at how comfortable it feels to focus on your fat forearms. Stepping off those scales for good is quite literally stepping out of your comfort zone. But just keep on breathing.

COCKTAIL FIVE:

No Longer Waiting to Exhale

This cocktail is a variation that often works well for athletes and others who want to keep their body and spine limber (yes, that's you). Because eliminating toxins is so important, this cocktail focuses on the exhale. When you don't exhale all the way, you leave stale and stagnant air in the body. This contributes to fatigue and any number of bodily ills. Remember diseases and microbes live in low-oxygen environments.

1. Stand up straight with your feet eighteen to twenty inches apart and toes pointed slightly outward.

2. Place your hands at your waist with palms inward and thumbs pointed toward the back.

3. Bend over from your hips as far as possible.

4. Exhale through your nose to a slow count of one through twelve while gradually pulling the abdomen wall inward as if you were deflating the abdomen.

5. Inhale deeply and fully through your nose to a slow count of twelve while expanding the abdomen.

6. Repeat steps four and five five times. Monitor inflating and deflating of your sides with your hands.

7. Hold your breath, and stand up slowly.

8. Exhale slowly.

9. Take a deep breath, and hold it at the core for a few seconds.

10. Relax and return to normal breathing.

Repeat this sequence three times.

THE OLIVE:

Trust Your Body

**''It is known that by the knowledge of
the breath, one gets good fruit
without much ado.''**
RAMA PRASAD, INDIAN YOGI AND
AUTHOR OF *THE SCIENCE OF BREATH*

The whole point of breathing is to learn to trust yourself, trust your body. Right now, you think of your body as a willful child that you must control, that you must keep very close tabs on.

As you breathe, keep paying attention to your body, notice its divinity. If you persist in seeing it as a big bag of lumpy flesh, ask yourself, "What investment do I have in staying lumpy?" And then, as you breathe into the vision, watch while it floats off into space like the helium balloon that you bought for your daughter at Wal-Mart. You know the one that she accidentally let go of, the one that flew off into the ionosphere while your daughter cried her sweet little heart out.

Now that that vision, thankfully, is gone, tell yourself this. My body is as smart as the dickens and it knows what to do without my help. Keep telling yourself that, if you'll just let it, your body will get rid of the weight without prompting of any kind from you. You've just got to surrender and say, "It's my turn."

When you refuse to work with your body by keeping tabs and counting calories you refuse to let your body change.

This may come as a shock to you—especially if you spend most of your waking moments silently carping about your ugly, cellulite-ridden body—but the normal state of your body is healthy. If you're overweight, some obstacle has gotten in the way. And I can guarantee you it didn't get there on its own. Somewhere along the way, you put up a roadblock.

Nobody bothered to mention that our bodies can regulate and heal themselves. Nowhere were we taught that our inner feelings and sensations are signals. On the contrary, we were taught to ignore these inner signals. We're brainwashed into listening instead to various outer authorities such as Dr. Atkins, Dr. Ruth, or, for that matter, me.

Sinclair Lewis was once asked to speak to a group of writing wanna-be's. He stepped to the podium with an air of authority and he asked how many of the participants would like to be writers. Every one of them proudly raised his or her hand. Lewis paused for a moment and then uttered these profound words: "Then why aren't you home writing?" And he walked off the stage.

He did come back and deliver a wonderful speech, but he made a point. Asking somebody else how to do something is blocking your own inner wisdom, thwarting the real answer. If you closed this book right now and started breathing and paying attention to your body, you'd be thin and enviously lithe within months. Quit searching for answers outside yourself.

Breathing will help you find yourself. It's the essential component. It will free you from the grasp of your little mind.

When you breathe, you'll also get in touch with the root problems that caused the weight in the first place. Now granted, such issues as self-protection, fear, and lack of discipline might not be the most pleasant emotions to face up to on a sunny Sunday afternoon. In fact, they are so painful that you may just need a bag of chocolate chip cookies to comfort yourself.

But by breathing, you can clear those feelings out of your body for good. Instead of making them disappear by stuffing them back down into your body, breathing can help free you from those feelings. Take a few big breaths into the physical sensation of any emotion and watch what happens. Many times, that's all it takes to move it out of your body. The unpleasantness of emotions comes from holding on to them like the ledge of a building you're about to fall off. When you participate with them, by breathing with them, you can rid yourself of them forever.

COCKTAIL SIX:

The Pump

Nike wasn't the first to invent the pump. In fact, this

exercise came from Thomas Hanna's book *Somatics,* which was written long before Michael Jordan ever stepped into a basketball shoe. As you begin to practice it, you'll become keenly aware of how much control you actually have over your breath. Do it once a day.

1. Lie on the floor with your knees slightly bent.

2. Start relaxing with a few deep belly breaths. Once you've gotten the hang of it, you're ready for the pump.

3. Inhale through your nose until your belly is round and full like a balloon.

4. Stop, hold your breath, and lock in that balloon of breath.

5. Now, while still holding your breath, flatten your back and belly, forcing the balloon of air upward into your chest, so that the chest swells up. Be careful not to let the air come out your nose or mouth.

6. Then flatten your chest, pushing the ball of air back down into the belly, while arching your back.

7. Continue this pumplike up-down movement until you need to take a breath. At first, this may be difficult to do, but as you gain breath control, you will be able to hold your breath longer, practice longer. Do the movement

vigorously and decisively like a piston, stroking upward and downward.

8. Stop and rest a moment. As you rest, breathing normally, can you feel more space for breathing in the abdomen and rib cage? Does the trunk seem less tight? Does everything in the trunk move more easily and softly as you breathe?

Every time you do this exercise, you will improve your breathing. You'll be taking in more air with less effort. The other thing this exercise does is diminish your hunger by forcing stomach acid down out of your stomach. Qi Gong practitioners swear by it.

THE OLIVE:

Be Bold and Brazen

> **''I never doubt myself. I just step back, take a deep breath, and figure out what I have to do.''**
> DWIGHT GOODEN, BASEBALL PLAYER

Sure, you can quietly hope to lose weight. You can poo-poo your fate, wishing in tragic silence that you'd sure appreciate being a tad bit skinnier. Or you can come right out and proclaim it with gusto: *"I am a thin and gorgeous human being. Look out world, here I come!!!"* This will let your body know that you are serious about being drop-dead gorgeous.

Whatever you do, refuse to put yourself down. Instead, become your own personal P.R. man. When you make comments like "I just look at a piece of apple pie and gain weight," your body listens and acts accordingly. Not only is your body recording every word, but your mental attitude becomes one of "I can't do it."

You can do it. Say it now.

There's a saying in the twelve-step program: "Fake it till you make it." Pretend that you are somebody you are fond of and wish to encourage. I doubt that you would look at a close friend and, in her presence, roll your eyes and snicker at her weight. I think you might come up with something along the lines of "Good job. Good for you. You're really trying."

If you refuse to say negative things about yourself for an entire three weeks, it will no longer feel comfortable. You'll actually feel weird making comments about the size of your body. But by then, it will have started to change, to have become what you have encouraged it to be.

COCKTAIL SEVEN:

Alternate Nostril Breathing

This one, which I've heard called "the five minute miracle," is great for balancing your nervous system. Not to suggest that your *nerves* might be shot, of course.

In each of our nostrils there are nerves that lead into the center of the brain. And as you undoubtedly know, the brain has two sides. There's the left side, the mechanical, calculating side that thinks in neat linear fashion. This is the side of choice in our Western Hemisphere, the side that says "be sensible," the side that works on known principles.

Then there's the right side, the creative, freewheeling, inspirational side, the side that invents, that says, "Wow, that's pretty neat," the side that refreshes and replenishes.

The yogis have found that there is a natural body rhythm. Every hour and a half or so, these sides of the brain alternate dominance. And, of course, your breath, the Sherlock Holmes of body function, will also reflect this. If the right side of the brain—the healing, resting side—is dominant, the left nostril will be dominant. If the left side of the brain—the mechanical calculator—is dominant, the right nostril will dominate. So . . .

1. Sit in a chair or on a comfortable mat on the floor with your back straight. Essentially, what you will be doing in this exercise is breathing in one nostril and out the other, then in the second nostril and out the first.

2. Using your index finger (either one) to hold the right nostril closed, breathe in with your left nostril to the count of six. Hold the breath for three counts.

3. Now, closing off the left nostril with your finger, release the right nostril and breathe out to the count of six.

4. Still closing your left nostril, breathe in with your right for six counts. Hold for three counts.

5. Then, closing off the right nostril, release the left nostril and breathe out to the count of six.

6. Repeat the entire sequence (steps two to five) six times.

By alternating the flow of air through your nostrils, you will experience an unbelievable sense of relaxation, and the balancing effect this will have on your brain will be miraculously tranquilizing.

You can do this exercise as often as you wish, but you should try to do it at least once a day during your week of experimentation. It wouldn't surprise me if you eventually add it to your daily repertoire. It is especially helpful if you think you're going to have a stressful day.

THE OLIVE:

Reset Your Life Enjoyment Thermostat

**"Deep, flowing breath is essentially
arousing and exciting."**
MICHAEL SKY, AUTHOR OF *BREATHING*

Do you remember the Robert De Niro film *The Mission,* where he played a fallen priest? I don't recall now whether he fornicated with somebody's wife or drank too much altar wine but whatever it was, his penance involved carting this incredibly heavy cross up a mountain. After several months of this grueling journey, his superior decided that he'd carried the cross far enough, he'd completed his penance. But De Niro, in his unbearable guilt, continued on lugging that cross, step after painful step.

Unfortunately that movie was more than a fantasy of the silver screen. Almost all of us carry some kind of cross, some kind of burden that, as far as everybody else is concerned, we could put down. But we're dogged in our determination to carry it ourselves—get your bloody hands off my cross. Deep down inside we believe we've done something terribly wrong, that God or our mother or maybe Sister Mary Margaret from second grade wants us to pay penance. We're not even exactly sure for what.

Perhaps that's why diets have appealed in the past. We believe that's all we deserve.

We deserve a lot more.

Remember the story of the prince who was turned into a frog? A wicked witch cast a spell on a handsome prince. He was stuck being an ugly, old frog until somebody decided to love him. Once the beautiful maiden kissed him, proving her love and friendship, he was magically restored to his rightful kingdom.

That's exactly what we human beings have done. Cast a spell over ourselves. Only it wasn't a witch at all. But our own failure to recognize our beauty. Our own inability to love ourselves.

Okay, so how do we do it?

When Trivial Pursuit first came out, I noticed a lot of answers were Reykjavik, Iceland—to what's the capital of Iceland, where was the current prime minister born, etc. So if I didn't know an answer to a question, I'd always pull out the standard. Although I have to admit Reykjavik, Iceland, got a few laughs when people wanted to know who had won the American League Batting Championship in 1977. In this book, however, if you get the one answer down, you'll be set. So what is the answer? All together now: *the breath*.

The best way to get past the crosses that you've unwittingly decided to bear is by breathing.

It's that simple. When we practice breathing, we increase our ability to enjoy life. Most of us have set our life enjoyment thermostat very low. We feel uncomfortable if we start having too much fun. It's not ladylike or gentlemanly.

What deep breathing does is retrain your nervous system to tolerate a higher charge of energy. If you practice it with any sort of regularity, you will find that you can feel good practically all the time. It'll be the crosses that don't feel natural.

That's why most spiritual traditions of the world encourage their devotees to practice breathing. People's faiths are strengthened when they feel good.

Experts tell us we could be breathing in seventeen pints of air per breath. Most of us settle for a measly two or three. Now, I don't know about you, but if somebody gave me the choice of one or two chocolate chip cookies or seventeen chocolate chip cookies, especially with the guarantee that the more I ate, the more weight I'd lose, I'd go for the seventeen.

Go for the breath.

COCKTAIL EIGHT:

The Goddess Breath

This is just about my favorite breath. It's imperative that you go outside to do it. Take off your shoes if at all possible.

The whole point is to feel your connection with Mother Earth and with all that's great and brilliant within you.

1. Stand with your feet apart about shoulder length.

2. Take a deep belly breath through your nose and really pull the strength of the ground up with it.

3. Feel your oneness with the planet. Feel yourself being grounded in the power of life.

4. Exhale with a deep, relaxing sigh through the mouth. Let go of all that excess emotional baggage you've been carting around. Forget it. It's not important.

5. If you want to, raise your arms over your head as you inhale and lower them as you exhale in sweeping, ballet-like movements. Remember to focus on the bigger picture. See yourself as a bigger piece of the whole.

This breath is very powerful at connecting with your spiritual side. It also helps you put things in their proper perspective.

THE OLIVE:

Make Your Motivation Exciting

"Breathwork allows the body's wisdom to heal itself."
JOHN CLARKE, M.D., PRESIDENT OF THE HIMALAYAN INTERNATIONAL IN-STITUTE OF YOGA SCIENCE

Most of us come up with diet goals like losing twenty pounds or shaving five inches off the waist.

This is not good enough. You need something that

will really fire you up. Something along the lines of looking so good that complete strangers approach you in elevators begging for dates. Something like Christie Brinkley's agent calling with the news that he's considering dumping her so he can make room for you on his list. You know what it is that trips your trigger. Think big. Think fantasy. Think dream come true.

Otherwise, your weight-change program is going to appeal to you about as much as lukewarm soap suds.

I mean who can wait to breathe when he or she knows it means being adored and envied by all. If your motivation is something like, "Well, my doctor said if I don't lose weight, I'll probably have gallstones," you are not as likely to stick with it. Remember this is FOR YOU and only you.

TAKE A BREATHER

CUTTINGLY CREATIVE VISUALIZATIONS

''THE MIND OF MAN IS CAPABLE OF ANYTHING...''
JOSEPH CONRAD

YOU may want to read any number of books that have been written about creative visualization. The basic idea is that you can change your life by visu-

JUMPSTART YOUR METABOLISM

alizing what you want to happen. Through mental imagery, you can literally revamp your physical body.

By forming a clear mental image of what you want to happen, you'll create that result. For example, if you'd like to lose weight in your thighs, you simply picture your thighs in the exact shape you'd like them to be. Eventually, by repeating the image, you'll manifest the desired thighs. You'll begin to act as though you have thin thighs, which will in turn create your thighs looking the exact way you want. Before long, your visualization will become a self-fulfilling prophecy.

Once I wanted to go to Australia because this chiropractor I had a crush on was moving there. I started visualizing it, imagining myself romping through the Sydney turf. I mean, I got really worked up over this movie in my mind. Within a week, the magazine *Modern Bride* called and assigned me a honeymoon story on Australia. Unfortunately, the chiropractor and I didn't repeat the honeymoon part of the visualization, but that's another story.

Some tips for increasing the effectiveness of visualization techniques:

1. Create a mental picture of anything you want to eliminate—say your flabby forearms. Visualize it in a form that makes sense to you.

2. Picture any steps you take as working. For

example, if you're doing exercises or using a piece of workout equipment, picture them working. Really *see* the weight falling off.

3. Imagine yourself healthy and beautiful. What would a person who looks like you want to look be doing? Picture yourself doing these things.

4. Keep in mind that the condition you want to eliminate is weak and can be easily changed.

5. Tell yourself that visualization and your mind are much more powerful.

And you don't have to depend only on your imagination. Create an actual picture of the new you. All you need are some photos of yourself, some photos of the body you want, a pair of scissors, and the willingness to be a little silly. After all, this weight-change business doesn't have to be so grim.

Just remember that visualizations work. Remember, your body is just a representation of your thoughts about yourself. Your physical self changes every day—really every minute—and by changing how you see your body, you can change your life.

Okay, so get out your scissors. Don't think, *This is ridiculous*. Starving yourself for two days and then the next day polishing off all the contents of your refrigerator is what's ridiculous!

COCKTAIL NINE:

Take 20

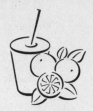

I learned this breath from Leonard Orr, the man who founded rebirthing. Leonard truly believes this one breath could save our planet. He's forever suggesting it to his students, government officials, boards of education, and anyone else who will listen.

This breath is more or less the foundation of rebirthing, which basically is learning to breathe energy along with air. This energy is the same energy that Indians call prana and Chinese call *chi*. It's really effective at getting your body and mind into harmony. I do this one every morning.

Leonard suggests doing connected breathing only once a day for the first week or so. After that, you can do it as often as it feels comfortable.

1. Alternate four inhales and four exhales through the nose without stopping between any one. It's natural to pause for a brief second or two between inhale and exhales, but with connected breathing the inhale and exhale flow into one another until you get the sensation of a circular river of energy.

2. Without breaking the connection, take one long inhale to the count of five and one long

exhale also to the count of five, still keeping the breath connected.

3. Do four sets of the five breaths—four shorts and one long—without stopping.

4. Most important, merge the inhale with the exhale so the breath is connected without any pauses—like a circle. All twenty breaths are connected in this manner so you have one series of twenty breaths with no pauses.

THE OLIVE:

Unlock the Issues Stuck in Your Tissues

''You are hedged in by energetic holding patterns that you know nothing about and that decided what you think life is like.''
JULIE HENDERSON, WRITER

When I was in grade school, a famous scientist discovered that every single event of our lives—the smells, the sights, the feelings—are faithfully recorded in our brains. He found out that if we probe certain parts of our brain, we can actually relive those memories.

We now know those same events are recorded in our body. The only problem is that a lot of our thoughts are submerged, locked away in some deep, dark cellular cellar.

Until we get in touch with some of these core issues, we will continue to be prisoners of our bodies.

This is why breathing—particularly rebirthing—is so important. As you begin to practice better breathing a couple of things will happen.

First, you'll become more aware of the thoughts that are affecting your body. Because so many of them are submerged—often because they're too uncomfortable— you can't really deal with them. But as you breathe, you become more in touch with all the emotions and thoughts that have been unwittingly running your life.

And the even better news is that by breathing into those painful feelings, you can move through them a whole lot faster. In fact, this could be the very best part of breathing. It moves energy around to heal those secret, hidden places in your cells. When you breathe you actually help to unloosen them and let them go.

Also, your cells will become more fluid. Remember the example of the glass blower? When you breathe, your cells heat up and become more pliable, more able to change. You can revamp the blueprint locked in your body. When you breathe, you can literally change the old thoughts and programming lodged in your cells and muscles.

Then you're free to create a different reality—different cells, a different neurochemistry.

COCKTAIL TEN:

The "I'm Stressed Out and Can't Take It Anymore" Breath

Okay, so you're having a good week. Congratulations! But it's still important to practice this cocktail so the next time you're *not* having a good week, you can remember to do it. This is also a great one to try before bedtime. Do this one as often as you like.

1. Stand up straight with your feet eighteen to twenty inches apart and toes pointed slightly outward. If you're doing this before bedtime, you can modify it by lying down.

2. Take five deep belly breaths through the nose.

3. Now, breathe in through your nose to any part of your body that feels tense or stressed out— like your shoulders, for example. Visualize the breath as a stream of light that's massaging and relaxing away tension.

4. As you exhale, imagine the tension streaming out your nostrils on each exhalation.

5. Let out a loud "Ahhh!" (yes, you can make a sound with your mouth closed) with each exhalation.

6. Make it rhythmic and smooth.

THE OLIVE:

*Get at Least Two Good Belly Laughs
a Day*

''Let your laughter fill the room''
MY HERO, VAN MORRISON

At the turn of the century, a doctor named Israel Waynbaum hypothesized that laughing gives the cells of the body an oxygen bath. This, he went on to say, elevates mood and induces a feeling of exuberance that persists long after the joke is over. He also said that chronic nonlaughers have the most breathing problems. So anytime the opportunity presents itself, have a good belly laugh. It will help you lose weight!

COCKTAIL ELEVEN:

Obstacle Breathing

This is another biggie with breathing coaches because by putting up an obstacle you make conscious contact with your breath. This particular version comes from Carola Speads's book, *Ways to Better Breathing*. By focusing on the out breath, more air goes out and when more air goes out, more air has to come in. Plus the simple act of pursing the lips forces you to breathe in a deeper, more diaphragmatic mode. Do this exercise ten times.

1. Find an everyday drinking straw.

2. Start paying attention to your "in breath" and "out breath."

3. Take a breath. Put the straw in your mouth and let the exhale come through the straw instead of through your nose. Be sure to raise the straw to your mouth rather than bending down toward it.

4. Pay attention to whether your exhalation passed through the straw of its own accord or whether you interfered. Try not to help at all. Don't blow, push, or force. You will gradually become aware of the extent of your interferences. Remove the straw just before the end of the exhale to let the rest of the air pass through your nose.

While this seems pretty benign at first, there are several benefits. By letting the air stream out as freely as possible through the straw, you actually expel more air than you ordinarily would. This is the key to increased inhalation. The pressure of the atmospheric air and the pressure of the air in the lungs have to equalize.

Furthermore, since the air can get out only slowly through the narrow straw, the diaphragm is forced to relax slowly rather than suddenly. Slow relaxation of the diaphragm improves muscle tone. As soon as your breathing apparatus is toned up, more efficient breathing follows.

It also gives you a simple and objective test to check the quality of your breathing. With the palm of your hand, feel the temperature of the first and last exhalation you let pass through the straw. You will discover the air at the end of your session is considerably warmer than your first exhalation. As air coming from the deeper part of your body is warmer, this indicates your breathing is deeper, less superficial than when you began.

THE OLIVE:

Have Faith

> **''Firmaments and planets have both disappeared, but the mighty breath which gives life to all things and in which all is bound up remained.''**
> VINCENT VAN GOGH

Changing your weight requires faith. Especially on those days when you look in the mirror and want to scream. Those days when you hate your hair, your eyes have bags, and your complexion is so splotched you might as well get out your eyebrow pencil and play dot-to-dot.

This is the time to remember the Nobel Prize—winning study about the cats who had been exposed to nothing but horizontal lines when they were kittens. After weeks of horizontal lines, they could no longer recognize vertical lines and literally bumped into chair legs. You've been practicing self-disapproval so long that you couldn't see your beauty if it stared at you from the pages of *Elle* magazine. You're an expert at picking out things you don't like. Everything else gets filtered out. Your beauty is not even recognizable—at least to you.

This is the time to exercise great discipline. You must guard against chastising yourself, feeling awful about who you are. What you put energy into will expand.

Lie to yourself if you must. Tell yourself you look beautiful. Pretend that Eileen Ford from the Ford Modeling Agency will be calling at any moment to offer you a job.

If necessary, don't look in the mirror again that day. Ask someone else to verify that your part is straight if need be. There's no reason to make yourself miserable.

Concentrate instead on the beautiful things about your personality. Your kindness, for example, or the extra hours you put in so a co-worker could have the day off.

This is also the time to go on a treasure hunt. Yes, you can always find something about your looks that you like. Your eyes, for example. Are they bloodshot? Good, you have beautiful, bright eyes. Do your ears stick out? Okay, at least you're not Alfred E. Neuman. Are your feet still size eight and a half, making shoes very easy to buy?

Focus on those little things, no matter how insignificant they might seem. What you focus on will expand.

By the same token, if there's a day you feel particularly thin (c'mon, there are plenty of those days and you know it), spend ample time enjoying it. Admire that beauty. It's only going to get better.

Learn to Love the Negatives

Quick, make a list of all the physical attributes you'd like to change. I know this won't be hard. Even beautiful fashion models claim they'd gladly alter certain features if they could.

Now take that list and endorse it. Tell those "ugly" parts, those features that you'd just as soon hide under a paper bag, that you love them. Give them a break. They're working as hard as they can. After all, they're just a translation of your thoughts.

Those fat forearms that embarrass you so much in the summer? Throw them a party. That double chin that makes turtlenecks your number-one fashion choice? Christen it gorgeous.

The more you accept these "ugly" traits, the freer they are to disappear. It's called the law of nonresistance. If you haven't put a lot of energy into hating them, they're free agents that can change quickly. If you detest them, hide them, deny them, they're going to stick around. After all, they're highly regarded—even if it's negative regard—guests. Whatever you resist, persists.

Your body is a mirror of your thoughts. If you've

exerted energy into hating your double chin, it's going to gladly follow your marching orders. Bless those ugly parts and you rob them of their ammunition. Send love and good will and you rob them of their power.

COCKTAIL TWELVE:

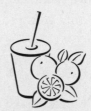

Mr. Clean

Ridding yourself of pollutants and tension is not always easy. In fact, when you first do this cleansing exercise and all the toxins become liberated from joints, muscles, and tissues, you may feel tired and headachy. Just know that it will pass and it's a normal sign of recovery from previously held body sludge. It's really a blessing in disguise. Do this sequence three times.

1. Sit in a comfortable chair.

2. Inhale deeply through the nose.

3. Exhale through a puckered mouth, shaped like an "o" as if you were blowing out a candle.

4. Repeat three times.

5. Let out a few deep sighs.

6. Repeat steps two through four, remembering to drop your shoulders.

7. Visualize yourself letting the air out of a tire.

THE OLIVE:

Are You Having Fun Yet?

"I do not normally like to hang around people who talk about slow conscious breathing; I start to worry that a nice long discussion of aromatherapy is right around the corner."
ANNE LAMOTT, AUTHOR OF *OPERATING INSTRUCTIONS* AND *BIRD BY BIRD*

In case you're not already, you should be pounding yourself on the back right now, giving yourself a big hug or maybe even an Academy Award. Really laying on the encouraging comments. Things like "Good for you. You deserve to be skinny and this is the time it's really going to happen."

Again, the first thing we have to change about this whole weight-loss business is the way we frame it in our minds. Think about it—the word diet, loss, starvation. I mean, who needs it?

What we want to do is turn the experience into something you can't wait to do, something you practically lose sleep over because you're so psyched to wake up and get started. This "program" you're embarking on is one of the most exciting things to ever happen in your entire life. You are going to finally realize goals and dreams you have wanted to realize for years. In other words, this is something that should trip your trigger. You are going to be skinny and beautiful and attractive strangers are going to be begging for your phone number. Whether or not you decide to give it to them is totally up to you.

Every time you think about being skinny, think about how much fun it is. Don't think about what a pain it is to get skinny. Or stay skinny. Because that's merely a thought. And it doesn't have to be true. Anymore than the thought that Tom Hanks is our best American actor is true. Some folks think it is, but many others don't. And neither is right. As Shakespeare once said, "Nothing is either good nor bad, only thinking makes it so." He probably said it a lot more poetically, but you get the gist. And this small change in attitude is absolutely essential.

COCKTAIL THIRTEEN:

Kapalabhati

In case you don't speak Sanskrit, Kapalabhati means skull-cleanser. It's an energizing breath that stimulates digestion and elimination. Do this once a day.

1. Sit in a comfortable position.

2. Do twenty deep belly breaths (see pages 23–24 for instructions).

3. Inhale fully through your nose.

4. Closing off your right nostril, expel short, forceful exhalations through the left nostril while pulling in your abdomen with each exhalation. You will experience a staccato exhalation until your lungs are fully emptied.

5. Repeat full inhalation and staccato exhalations ten times. Any inhalation between staccato exhales should be involuntary and passive.

6. Inhale fully through the nose.

7. Exhale fully through the nose.

8. Inhale to about three-quarters of your lung capacity and hold as long as comfortable, then exhale.

9. Repeat steps four to eight through the right nostril.

10. Finish by repeating steps four to eight simultaneously through both nostrils.

THE OLIVE:

Things to Do Besides Obsess About Your Weight

> **"We can learn to use the breath as a Geiger counter to sense, locate, and define our experience."**
> DONNA FARHI, AUTHOR OF
> *THE BREATHING BOOK*

You've probably heard that old Bible verse about man not living on bread alone. For those of us on a diet, this really doesn't compute. Pretty much everything in life as we know it revolves around the next meal—what it's going to be, what time we're going to eat it, how many calories it's going to have.

Unfortunately, this is not a very good life strategy.

Deepak Chopra, who wrote a book called *Perfect Weight,* pointed out that it *is* possible to get sustenance from other things besides food. Like . . . oh, you know, having a good time. Or doing something constructive for yourself. When life-sustaining nutrition is received from sources other than food, the need to eat is diminished.

Chopra cited a lab study where seven groups of rabbits were all fed the same amount of cholesterol. One group seemed immune and actually thrived on the high doses of cholesterol. Upon further investigation, it was discovered that the lab assistant feeding that particular group spent a lot more time with his bunnies, talking to them, stroking them, singing them lullabies. These bunnies were actually "fed" by kindness and love.

One of the ways I "feed myself" is to go on adventures. They don't have to be big ones—I mean how many times can you climb Pikes Peak in the course of the average lifetime—but something that shakes me out of my normal rut, some little activity that reminds me that life is more than a piece of cherry cheesecake.

If you're one of these people who thinks of little else but food and all its possibilities, then you need to—how can I say this politely—"get a life."

Thinking about your weight and your diet is not exactly a productive way to spend your time—at least not more than say an hour a month. Next time you're starting to wonder how many fat grams are in that box of Twinkies Hi-Ho's, stop, breathe, and try something else.

From now on, your only responsibility is to enjoy life. Get a hobby. Fall in love with yourself. Write a screenplay. "Skip to my Lou."

I don't care what you do. Just do not think about weight or food or calories or fat grams or cellulite or . . .

Let it go. Trust the universe.

RECOMMENDED RESOURCES

Now that you've discovered the power of breath (and are undoubtedly wondering, "Where have you been all my life"), you're probably eager to learn more. I know I will always consider myself a student of breathing, a rapt pupil in constant awe of its amazing power. The more I study and use breathing, the more I discover how vast and deep is its potential.

Here are some books I highly recommend.

The Art of Breathing by Nancy Zi. Coming from a professional singer, this book is chockful of breathing exercises—must be at least a hundred of them.

Birth Without Violence by Dr. Frederick LeBoyer.

Breathing by Michael Sky. A poem as much as a book. You'll never feel the same about your breath again.

The Breathing Book by Donna Farhi. If you're a visual person, this is the book for you. There are more than seventy-five photos and illustrations to help illuminate the concepts. Farhi is a yoga teacher and a registered movement therapist.

Breathplay by Ian Jackson. Fitness expert Jackson has lectured on his unique breathing methods for many years. His focus is on the exhale.

The Breath Connection by Robert Fried, Ph.D. A good primer to the problems caused by faulty breathing complete with exercises for overcoming them.

Celebration of Breath by Sondra Ray. Although it's a little disjointed, this book gives a good understanding of what Sondra calls rebirthing.

Conscious Breathing by Gay Hendricks. This book is a must for anyone interested in breathing. After twenty years of counseling, lecturing, and writing books, Hendricks really knows his stuff.

The Oxygen Breakthrough: 30 Days to an Illness-Free Life by Dr. Sheldon Saul Hendler. For a convincing argument on the health hazards of not breathing properly, be sure to read this one. Hendler is a biochemist and M.D.

The Tao of Natural Breathing by Dennis Lewis. This is an excellent book that focuses on what the breath can teach you about the body.

Take a Deep Breath by Dr. James E. Loehr and Dr. Jeffrey A. Migdow. If you're interested in an overview, this would be a good book to try. It's particularly helpful for athletes.

Total Breathing by Phillip Smith. One of the first books written on breathing, it is filled with lots of good breathing techniques. When he was laid up with an injury, this former athlete decided to develop his breathing power.

Unlimited Power by Anthony Robbins. This one hit the bestseller list a few years ago. If you missed it, check out the chapter on energy.

Ways to Better Breathing by Carola Speads. If anyone knows the breath, it's Speads, who worked in private breath practice for many years.

May the breath be with you . . .

. . . with all its accompanying peace,
passion, and prosperity.

PAM GROUT

INDEX

goddess breath, 148–49
Goode, Tom, 41
guided tour, 127–30

Hanna, Thomas, 131, 141
hara, 124
health, 54, 68–69, 90, 108–10
heart, 87, 96
Hendler, Sheldon Saul, 108–10
Hendricks, Gay, 14, 105, 107, 128
hormones, and exercise, 34–35
hydrocarbons, 64

illness, 54, 68–69, 90, 108–10
immune system, 69
insulin, 82
intestines, and muscle
   contractions, 34

kapalabhati, 164–65
kung fu breath, 123–25

lactic acid, 72
Lamb, Lawrence, 18, 63
laughter, 157
LeBoyer, Frederick, 54–55
liquid, processing of, 18–19
Loehr, James, 105
lungs, 87, 89, 129
   capacity of, 21, 98
lymphatic system, 81

memory, 154–55
menopause, 110
metabolism, 74–83
   anaerobic, 67–68
   basal, 61, 78
   and body heat, 78–80
   and burning food, 77–78
   changes in, 29–30, 74
   defined, 78
   and diets, 61
   efficiency of, 76, 78
   and exercise, 23, 72

and oxygen intake, 30, 76,78
   and weight gain, 29
mindfulness, 102–3, 131–32
muscles, and adrenaline, 34

nerve receptors, 34–35
neurochemistry, 131, 155
neurolinguistic programming, 50
nonresistance, law of, 161
norepinephrine, 82
nose:
   alternate nostril breathing,
      143–45
   breath strips on, 30
   vs. mouth breathing, 27–28

obstacle breathing, 157–59
olives, 116
   #1: make breathing fun, 121–
      23
   #2: Albert Einstein theory of
      weight loss, 125–27
   #3: put a lock on it, 130–32
   #4: trash bathroom scales,
      134–36
   #5: trust your body, 138–40
   #6: be bold and brazen, 142–43
   #7: reset enjoyment
      thermostat, 146–48
   #8: make motivation exciting,
      149–50
   #9: unlock the issues, 154–55
   #10: get daily belly laughs, 157
   #11: have faith, 159–62
   #12: having fun yet?, 163–64
   #13: things to do, 166–67
Orr, Leonard, 153
oxidation, 19, 72, 76
oxygen, 100–111
   allotropic, 69
   benefits of, 100–110
   consumption of, 18
   deprivation of, 21, 44, 48–49
   and digestion, 33